Beautiful Hair
by Suga

Beautiful Hair
by Suga

Suga with Alexandra Penney

designed by
Constance von Collande

Random House
New York

**Photographs
by Gordon Munro,
illustrations
by the author**

Library of Congress Cataloging in Publication Data

Suga, Yusuke.
Beautiful Hair by Suga.

1. Hairdressing.   2. Hair—Care and hygiene.
I.   Penney, Alexandra, joint author.   II. Title
TT957.S82   646.7'242   79-4772
ISBN 0-394-50750-9

Manufactured in the United States of America
24689753
First Edition

Acknowledgments

There was no possibility of this book without the help of my dear friend Alexandra. I really thank her from the bottom of my heart.

I would like my two other friends and collaborators, Constance von Collande and Gordon Munro, to know how much I have appreciated their patience, kindness and, above all, their talent.

Thanks to Yvonne Larchian for her diplomacy, tact and helpfulness in every way.

Thanks to my good friends who gave so much of their valuable time and whose most beautiful faces appear in this book. I love you all and you will understand why I must list your names in alphabetical order:

Candice Bergen, Faye Dunaway, Karen Graham, Dorothy Hamill, Margaux Hemingway, Lauren Hutton, Beverly Johnson, Marie Osmond, Jane Lee Salmons, Sayoko.

So many models and actresses were kind enough to give freely of their time. I give you many thanks and much appreciation:

Sara Abrell, Susan Bearden, Kate Capshaw, Caroline, Holly Colburn, Toni De Marco, Emma, Jerry Hall, Rosie Hall, Paula Holland, Jennifer Mann, Marie Louise, Maura, Ella Miloszlwska, Jeanne Ongaro, Ritsuko, Rene Russo, Marina Schiano, Diane St. Cyr, Constance Walter, Leslie Winer.

The following friends helped mentally, emotionally, physically—and every other way:

Dick Avedon, Paul Finkelstein, Cathy Hardwick, Hanae Mori, Carl Morton, Sadao, Armand St. Gelais, Yukiko Sakai, Norman F. Stevens, and all my assistants.

To Sakiyo Suga

Contents

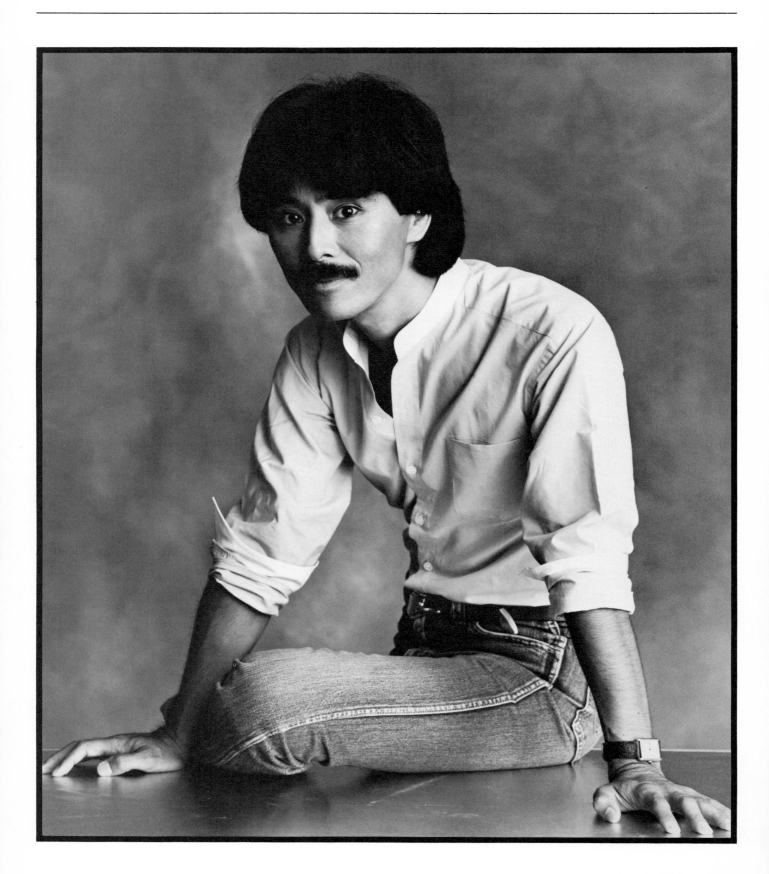

Suga on Suga

At the age of twenty-one I packed my electric rice cooker and one suitcase and left my native Japan for America. It had suddenly dawned on me that everyone in Japan who was seriously interested in fashion—people like Kenzo and Issey Miyake—had gone West, and although at the time I knew no English, I knew when I arrived in America that I would stay.

I began my career in the States by asking people who knew about hair which was the best salon in New York. Many people told me "Kenneth's," so I was determined to work there.

On January 2, 1966, I finally managed to obtain an interview at Kenneth's. When I arrived at the salon, I was dazzled by the lavishness of the décor, in such contrast to the simplicity of Japanese salons. At 11 A.M. I began to set and comb the three test models they had provided me, and at 3 P.M. I finished. Although I didn't meet Kenneth that day, they hired me for $100 a week!

I stayed three years at Kenneth's as his personal assistant, setting his clients' hair and learning his techniques. On my daily client sheets I found names like Jacqueline Kennedy, Barbra Streisand, Diana Ross, Lee Remick and Elizabeth Ashley. Kenneth took me on my first private jet ride to a client on Cape Cod and then to the *Mike Douglas Show* in Philadelphia. After that he sent me to do photographic shootings with *Town and Country, Harper's Bazaar,* and then *Vogue.* The experience with magazine and fashion photography was what I had been looking for, as I had always been interested in free-lance work, and had been one of the first hairdressers in Japan to free-lance for magazines. So within half a year of coming to the States I was doing magazine

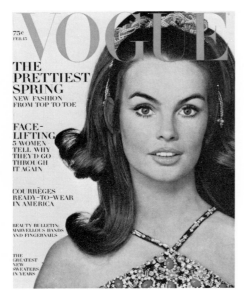

Jean Shrimpton
trend-setter of the sixties,
one of the first supermodels.
Hair: Suga. Photo: Penn

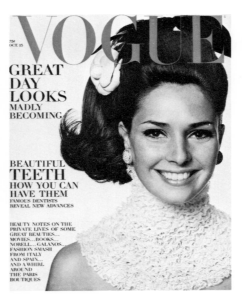

Jennifer O'Neill
model in the sixties and
movie star in the seventies.
Hair: Suga. Photo: Bailey

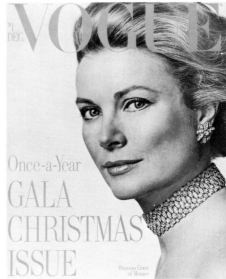

Princess Grace
epitomizes the ideal of
classical charm and elegance.
Hair: Suga. Photo: Avedon

assignments and working with America's beautiful people. But I was beginning to have a major problem with time. I was very often out of the salon on location with magazines for several days and I was also having to take private clients on weekends and after-salon hours.

I was caught between the magazines needing me and my clients, who also needed me. I ended up trying to please both sides and was really doing two jobs at once. I felt if I kept on that way one or the other would suffer—and so would I. So exactly three years to the day that I started at Kenneth's, I left, to concentrate on free-lance work while keeping some of my clients. But I will never forget the opportunities Kenneth gave me.

After I left I continued working with magazines. One of my private clients, Mrs. John Sherman Cooper, a leader of Washington society, flew me down to the capital once a month to do her hair. Mrs. Cooper's circle of friends was large and included many senators' wives, and after a while on my Washington visits Mrs. Cooper's room turned into a beauty salon, with Mrs. Coo-

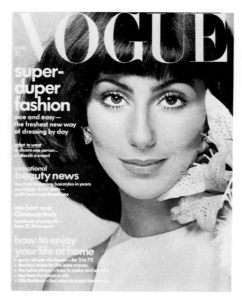

Cher
vitality and energy, an
upbeat woman all the time.
Hair: Suga. Photo: Avedon

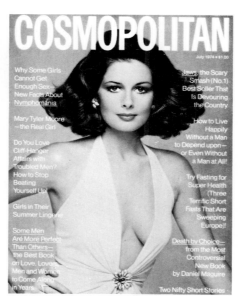

Cristina Ferrare
beautiful blue eyes set
against wonderful brown hair.
Hair: Suga. Photo: Scavullo

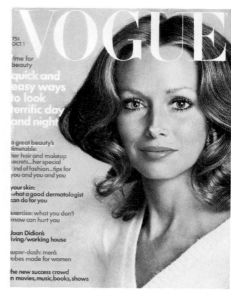

Karen Graham
a perfect face that
launches great cosmetics.
Hair: Suga. Photo: Avedon

per's secretary taking appointments. (Today, many of these clients take day trips to my New York salon.)

Life as a free-lancer is exciting but hectic, and I found that I missed working in a real salon. So in the fall of 1972 I opened my own salon in a brownstone on East Seventieth Street. I had specifically chosen a location in a quiet neighborhood away from most hair salons so that the ambience of my salon would be both relaxed and luxurious. I felt that Japanese style and service would be well received in New York, and I traveled back to Japan to find young Japanese hairdressers to work and train with me. I brought two young men and a young woman with me, and with them, along with several others, I opened the new salon. One client described the atmosphere of the salon as a "mixture of Japanese serenity and American efficiency."

Although the salon was successful and allowed me to continue doing some free-lance work for magazines, cosmetic houses and television, my interests began to conflict, and it was at this time that I had the enticing offer from Bergdorf Goodman's on

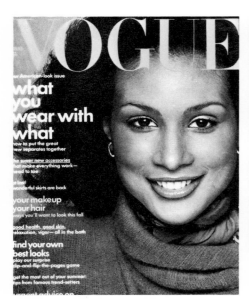

Beverly Johnson
has glamour galore, vitality, and a sure sense of style.
Hair: Suga. Photo: Scavullo.

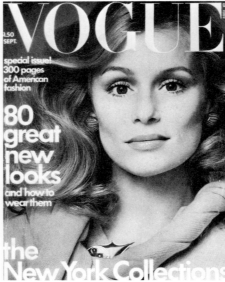

Lauren Hutton
model and actress, beautiful, interesting, intelligent, witty.
Hair: Suga. Photo: Avedon.

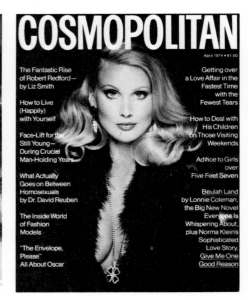

Cathy Spiers
has fabulous hair, flawless skin and magnetic eyes.
Hair: Suga. Photo: Scavullo.

Fifth Avenue, one of the city's oldest and most elegant stores, to move my operation over there. After giving it some thought, I accepted because day-to-day business problems would be handled more efficiently, and I would be freer to do my out-of-salon fashion work in a less frenzied manner.

I feel that doing both salon and free-lance work is challenging and seems to be the right mix for me. I enjoy doing photographs of shootings and advertising and television work; having stars as clients gives me an opportunity to travel, which I also love. Although America is my home, I hope to be able to cross the Pacific often because the young people in Japan have a great deal of interest in fashion and hair, and I would like to put some energy there.

I need a fast pace and I like changes. Although I wouldn't give up my free-lance work, I always want to stay in touch with the public—working on a personal level with any woman who wants me to cut and style her hair.

SUGA

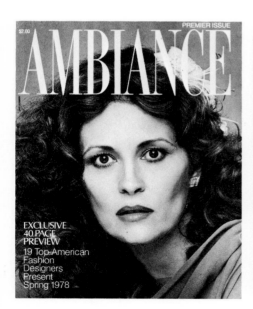

Faye Dunaway

superstar, one of the
great beauties of our time.
Hair: Suga. Photo: Priggen.

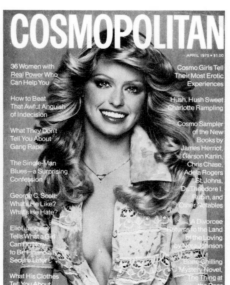

Farrah Fawcett

fabulous mane of hair
is her trademark.
Hair: Suga. Photo: Scavullo.

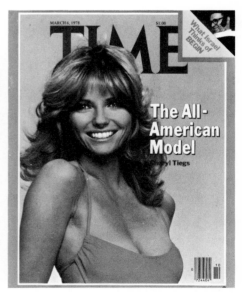

Cheryl Tiegs

a high-voltage smile and
All-American good looks.
Hair: Suga. Photo: Hiro.

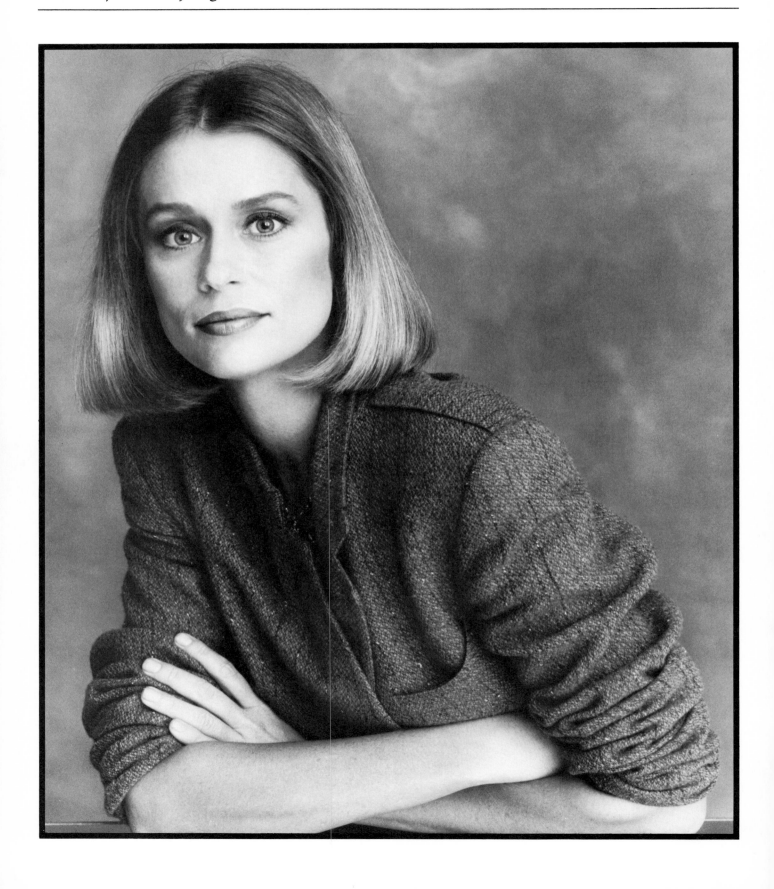

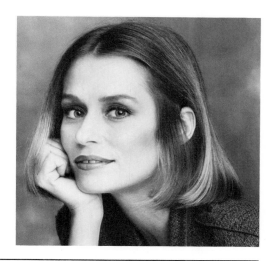

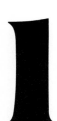

Who's in control, you or your hair?

We have certainly done some odd things to hair. I remember when teen-age girls, in the not so long-ago past, ironed their hair with real irons and ironing boards so they could have stick-straight hair. Women who were otherwise wise slept in painful rollers, incurring headaches and the wrath of their husbands for the sake of a "bouffant" look, or they spent hours under the dryer with complicated sets and even more complicated comb-outs. More time was spent stripping the hair of all its God-given color and then coating it with hues that nature herself would

Above, left: Lauren Hutton, actress with a very special face and personality. Her fine hair is blunt-cut all in one length for versatility. *Make-up: Sandy Lintner.*

have considered crazy and impossible. Then there were some women who, upon returning with a "style" from the beauty salon, wanted to preserve the hairdresser's work hair for hair until the next salon visit, so they covered their heads with all sorts of apparatuses at night and never dared lift a finger, much less a comb, lest the precious style be disturbed. Much of the madness about hair in those days stemmed from fashion. Those were the days when designers and beauty experts decreed a new look or style each season, and women willingly followed their pronouncements. One fashionable woman I know confessed to me that in order to achieve the look in vogue at the time, she went to one hairdresser who cut the hair at the nape of her neck "just so" and to another hairdresser who cut the rest of the hair on her head. Today, when I think of the time—not to mention the money—expended on this double haircut, I think it's a clear example of the hair controlling its owner and not the other way around, which is the way I feel it should be.

Some women are really afraid of their hair. They actually let it dominate their thoughts. Many of us, men as well as women, feel that we don't really look well unless our hair is "right," and in a way we can become obsessed with it. It's really not possible for hair to look "perfect" or "right" all the time. Hair changes day by day. First of all, it grows—and that changes it. Second, physical and hormonal changes, the way you sleep, what you eat, how you feel, can very much affect the way hair looks and falls. Third, stress and anxiety, which seem to be basic elements of life today, also contribute to limp, lusterless, bodyless hair. You must realize that hair is a changeable element and, as such, cannot consistently look "perfect" every day.

I don't think that hair should look perfect, anyway. A well-known artist once said that if something was perfect it was ultimately boring. The small imperfections, a wisp out of place, a curl that won't behave, a wave where you don't want it, can

Right: One of the best easy-care styles comes from naturally wavy air-dried hair.

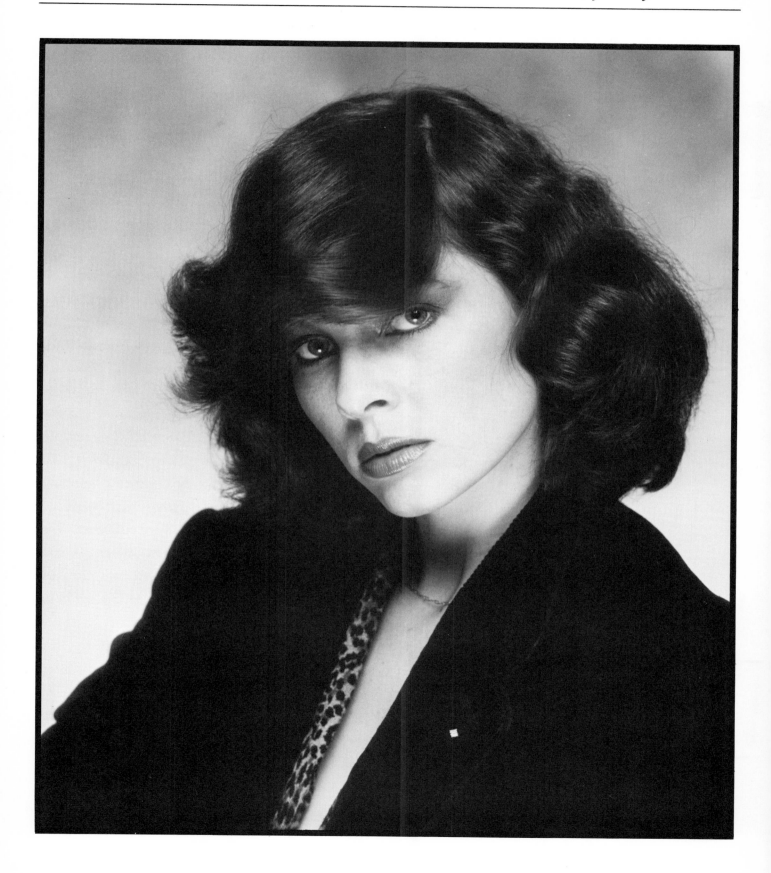

make your hair look human and make you look more interesting. Today we are involved with a natural look, and I think that this kind of free, healthy attitude is good for all of us and it is especially good for hair. You must learn to live with what you've got naturally, and learn to cope with the hair you've been endowed with. Your hair can and should look attractive, be easy to care for, take a minimum of time—and that's it. Then you should forget it.

Some of you may have to adjust your thinking to accept the idea of simple, easy-to-care-for hair. What I mean by this is, you should make the most of what you have and not ask too much from your hair. It should be *your* decision if you want to take extra time to do a special hair style for a special occasion, but generally speaking, your hair should really require a minimum of time and thought to look its best. In the next chapter there are some simple tests that allow you to evaluate your hair type; once you understand what it can and cannot do, then you are on the road to being in charge and finding a look that works for you.

Another interesting psychological aspect was pointed out to me by a beauty editor of *Glamour* magazine. She told me that when women have had make-overs—that is, when they have had their hair and make-up and clothes planned for them by the *Glamour* editors and fashion and beauty experts—most of them go back to their original hair and make-up look. Although many women believe that they want to change to something different and that they want an authority like a hairdresser or a fashion editor to tell them what looks best on them, when the big change is finally made, they are uncomfortable with it and return to their previous style. I think the reason why this happens is that you can never really tell another person what is best for her. However, you *can* work with another person—if she is willing—to come up with a look that is comfortable and fits her personality and life style. This is especially true for hairdressers, I think. We must work with the clients, not just force our own ideas on them.

Many women come to me tired and bored with their hair style and they ask for something different—immediately! Sometimes when a woman has had an upsetting change in her life she wants to dramatically change her hair style—and then she regrets it. A

UNCONTROLLABLE IMPULSES
Bianca Jagger usually wears her hair rolled, in a chignon, or just down. I went to visit her in her hotel to roll her hair, but she wanted to have her hair cut short—she was adamant about it. Of course I could have cut her hair in her room, but when a woman all of a sudden wants to have her hair cut short there's usually a story behind it. I therefore suggested that she come to the salon the next day so I could cut it properly with a mirror and shampoo—she never showed up!

hairdresser is neither a magician nor a psychologist. He can cut hair and he can recommend different hair styles, but basically he must work with what's there—and what's there is exactly what a woman has on her head. A hairdresser should also have some idea of what's *in* the client's head as well. And for this to happen, a woman must communicate with her hairdresser as to what she wants, what her life is like and what she feels comfortable with. What I have found is that women are often apprehensive about going to a new hairdresser, and at the same time they expect miracles from him.

You can cut, color, permanent, straighten, set, style and condition hair. A good cut is necessary, and beyond that I advise keeping the other processes to a minimum if you possibly can. This way you can forget about your hair and concentrate on other things that are far more important!

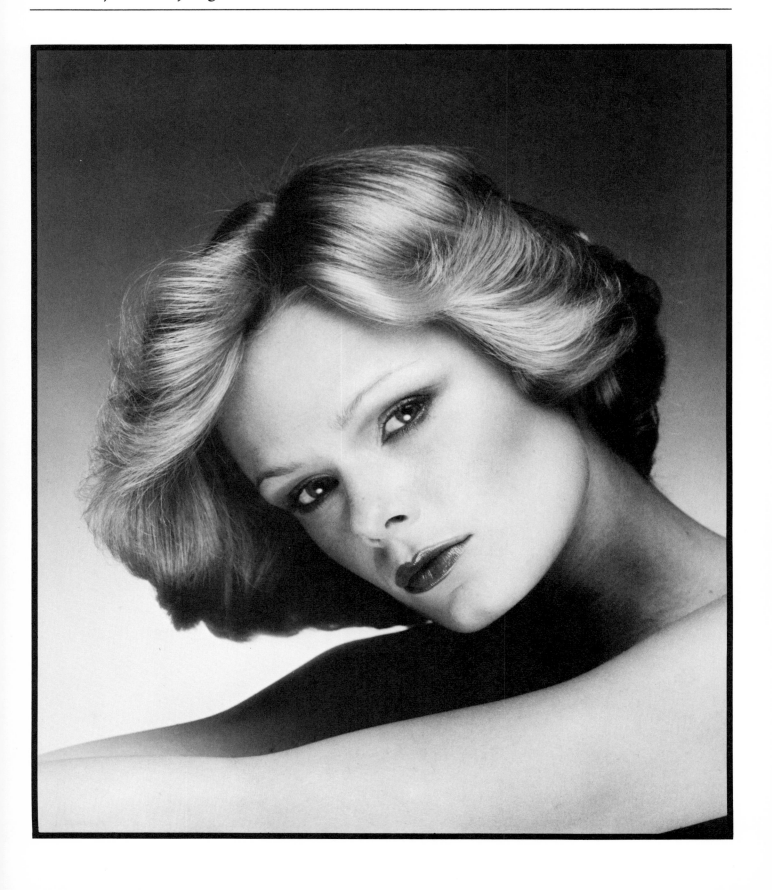

2

Which hair looks are right for you

There are really no rules about hair. Someone might have told you "you cannot have long hair," or "you cannot have short hair." This is simply not true. What *is* true, and more to the point, is that there are certain types of hair which usually don't work at certain lengths and in certain styles. Coarse, straight hair should not be worn extra short (it will probably tuft out all over the head), and very fine hair should probably not be worn long because it will not swing right. But these are very general rules and I have seen them broken with beautiful results.

Left: Know your hair type; texture and degree of curl are crucial factors.

We all see charts of hair styles that go with oval faces, round faces, square faces. Forget these rules too. The shape of your face has nothing to do with whether you can wear long or short hair.

It used to be thought that an oval face was the most desirable shape to have. I don't believe that anymore. An unusual shape of face with the right style of hair is far more interesting than an oval that has everything "perfect" about it—including the hair.

I say that there are no rules, but I do feel strongly that there are some guidelines about hair. The most important is that *you must learn to live with your hair type.* Almost no one I know is satisfied with hers. It seems that the hair on another's head is always better than your own, especially the hair on the models. But please don't forget that a model in the glossy pages of *Vogue* and other fashion magazines or a model in a television commercial has had her hair done especially for the photo session or the TV camera, and that the hairdresser is standing no more than three feet away from her, brush in hand or blowing her hair with a fan so it moves perfectly while she's posing for the shot.

Your hair type is based on texture (coarse, medium or fine) and degree of wave. You probably know what hair type you have, but if you don't you might try these two quick tests.

Drying-time test: for texture

First, shampoo your hair and towel-dry it in a normally heated room. *Fine hair* should air-dry naturally in fifteen to twenty minutes, *medium hair* takes thirty to forty-five minutes, and *coarse hair* takes more than forty-five minutes. If you use a hand dryer to blow-dry your hair, *fine hair* will take five to eight minutes, *medium hair* eight to fifteen minutes, and *coarse hair* fifteen minutes or more. Very long or short hair are exceptions.

Wave test: for degree of curl

Shampoo your hair and comb it with a wide-tooth comb; first making a center part. Comb the wet hair straight down on either side of the center part. Then push the hair several times with the palms of your hands to form waves. If the diameter of a wave is less than ½ inch, your hair is considered frizzy; if from ½ inch to 1½ inches, your hair is curly; if from 1½ to 2½ inches, it is wavy. You must do this test right after a shampoo, as the degree of curl shows most when hair is wet.

Also remember that when you have longer hair, the weight of the hair tends to straighten the curl, so you may have basically curly hair which hangs straighter because it is longer. Also, sometimes you will find more curl in your hair after it has been cut. Again, this is because the weight of the hair tended to straighten it.

Another thing to look for in your hair is the way or pattern in which it grows. If hair is combed the way it grows, it lies flat to the head, but if you go against its natural growth pattern, it will stand up. You can use this growth pattern to give shape and volume to your hair. For example, I have a cowlick in the back of my head, but I comb the hair there in the opposite direction. This makes the hair stand up slightly and gives me the volume I need to make a rounded shape at the back of my head.

At times the way hair grows can be a problem. If you want your hair to lie flat or to wave in a certain direction, you may be literally going against the grain, but this can usually be tamed by blow-drying, setting or a permanent.

"which style is right for me?"

This is the second most often asked question (the first is "Which shampoo should I use?" and I'll come to that later). My answer is that you can't remove the head and neck from the rest of the body. It's much the same idea as trying to choose shoes without seeing the dress that they are to be worn with—you need to balance heel height and shape with the length and cut of the dress. In the same way, balance and proportions of the head to the entire body are always important, and of course, this relates directly to the hair. Many a client comes to the salon and considers a hair style according to her face only. You must think in terms of your body, too. I don't suggest that somebody wear long masses of hair if she is very tiny or that she try to have a small head of hair if she is very tall with broad shoulders. Again, I must stress that this does not always hold true, but much more often than not, it does.

Even the color of your hair may affect the proportions of your body. Medium to dark hair is more noticeable than lighter shades. Usually medium to dark hair should not be longer than five inches below the shoulder line because when you stand up you may look top-heavy, especially from behind. In any case, a big head of hair (either light or dark) usually upsets the natural proportions of the body, so if you have long hair, please remember to show somewhere the natural shape of your head at the top or on the sides. By doing this, you define the line of your head and keep the head/body proportions in balance. If your face is very narrow and long, you don't need volume on the top—you probably need width more than height. And if your face is wide or roundish, you probably need more volume on top and less at the sides. These are very general rules, and it's best to discuss these ideas with your hairdresser with a mirror in hand so you can see the back and sides of your head. It's also a good idea, when discussing or considering a hair style, to stand up and evaluate it in terms of your whole body, not just your face.

You must choose a style that is geared to the way you live. If you have four children and are a busy mother or if you are busy with a job, don't be a slave to your hair, too. You shouldn't think of an everyday hair look that requires setting. If you're very active, you probably would do better with short hair, but if you like it long it should be long enough to pull or pin back.

Dorothy Hamill

Ice skater Dorothy Hamill's cut was a result of function as well as style. She could not wear hair around her face or bangs longer than eyebrow length (so that she could see), and her hair also had to move well.

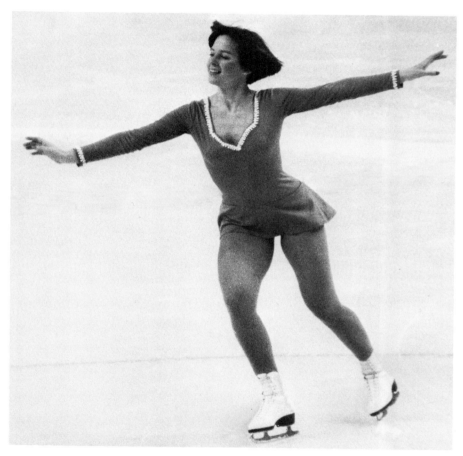

Think in terms of your occupation. Dancers, tennis players and office workers ask me for looks based on their activities. If, for example, you spend time typing and are always looking down, long hair can be irritating. I would suggest short hair, or hair long enough so that it can be tied back or anchored with combs.

Please note that when you play sports you should forget about hair styles and a "done" look. Just go with whatever is strictly functional—short, slicked back or long and tied—whatever lets you run fastest or win the game most easily.

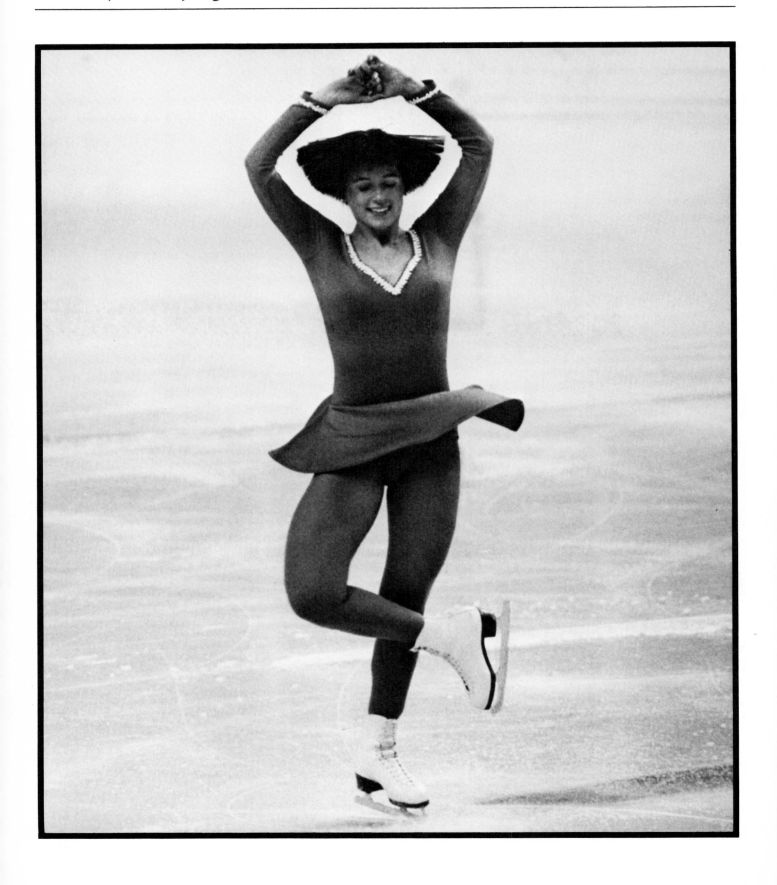

CHAMPIONSHIP HAIR

I have been cutting Dorothy Hamill's hair since the year before she won the Olympic gold medal. I had been doing another skater and Dorothy had wanted me to cut her hair, but I had been so overbooked that she couldn't get an appointment for six months. Finally her father called me from Canada and explained that a very important championship was coming up and could I please do Dorothy's hair. It turned out that she had only one free day in New York and that was my day off, but since I like sports and had heard she was going to be in the Olympics, I opened up the shop and cut her hair.

She let me do anything I wanted with her hair as long as it didn't fall in her eyes. We worked on the style several times, and then, two weeks before the Olympics, I cut it so that it would be a perfect length in fourteen days' time.

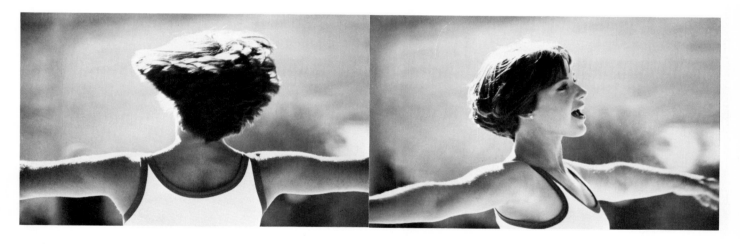

I've been cutting her hair ever since except for one time when a sponsor for shampoo insisted that she have a different hairdresser when she was making a commercial. A week later she called me from Philadelphia, nearly in tears, and told me, "My hair doesn't move anymore," so I was on the train to Philadelphia in three hours.

After Dorothy won the gold medal she has been on the road constantly and is not in New York as frequently as before. Now every eight weeks I fly to her anywhere in the country and give her a cut—thanks to Dorothy I've seen Kansas City, Cincinnati, Detroit, Buffalo and Atlantic City.

Above: Dorothy says she really can't skate well if her hair isn't cut properly. Photos above: Gideon Lewin. Photos left page, and page 17: UPI

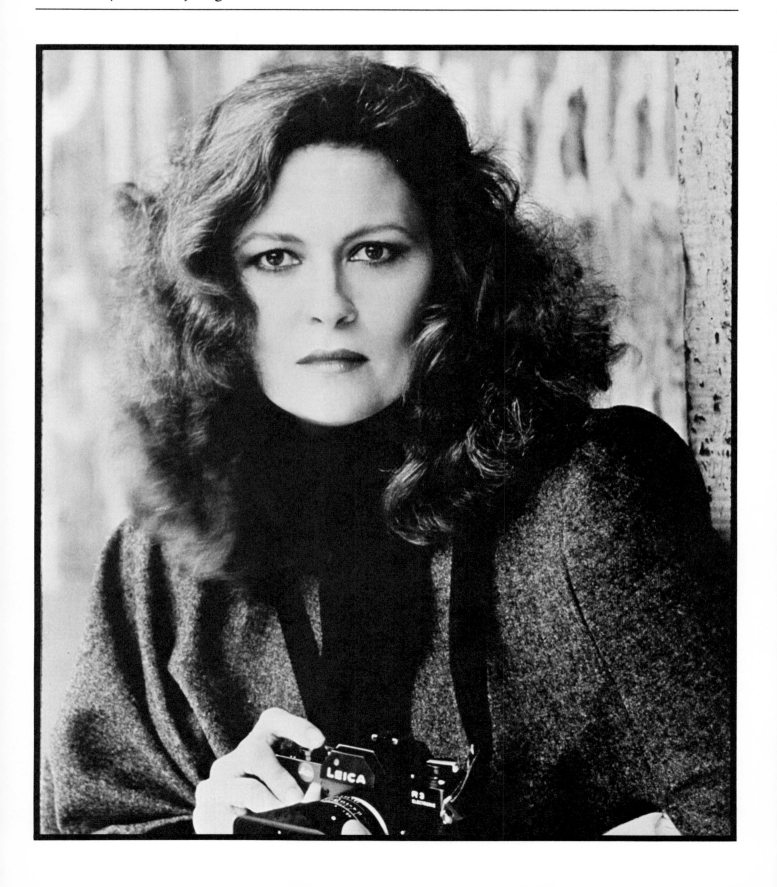

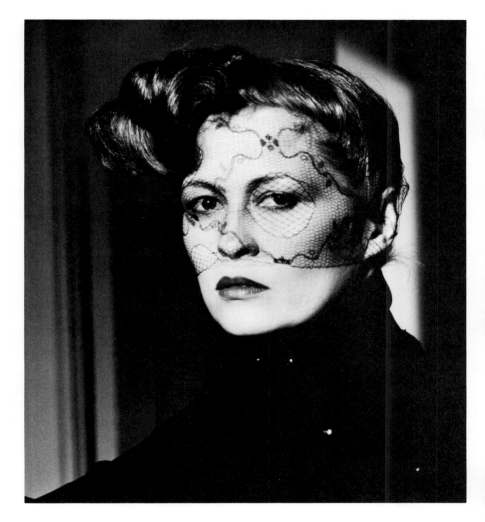

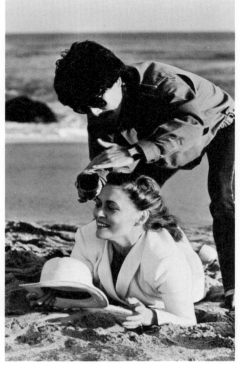

Faye and I have to work under any conditions and in the most awkward positions. *Above:* at the beach. *Below:* in her bathroom.

Faye Dunaway

Faye Dunaway is a good example of a woman who never forces her hair to do anything it wouldn't do naturally. She has medium-fine hair that is between curly and wavy. It's quite beautiful when she just washes it and lets it dry naturally. She has a trim once every eight weeks, and most of the time she styles it herself into a simple, natural-looking twist. For screen appearances, she likes a more finished look, and her hair is often set so that it keeps its style all day long.

Opposite: Faye's hair is naturally wavy and medium fine. From *Eyes of Laura Mars.* Photo: Terry O'Neill. *Above:* More on veils, p. 124. Photo: Kurigami. Courtesy of Seibu. Art direction: Ishioka.

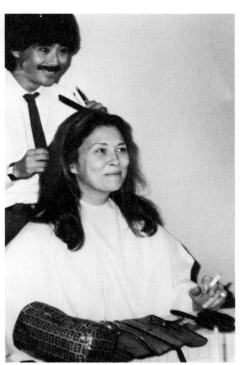

Candice Bergen

Candice Bergen has medium-textured, straightish hair and often goes for hair-conditioning treatments to keep it in the best condition possible. She has tried many different styles, but she looks best with longish hair naturally down or pulled back. Anything in between these two looks doesn't really seem "right" on her.

Hair fashion changes, of course, but not as quickly as clothes, and the newest styles in magazines do not become widespread for a long time. I often say to friends and clients, "Be brave and try

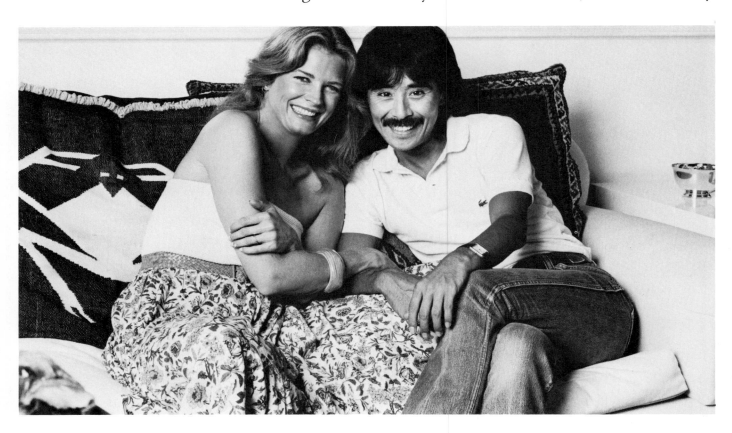

Above and right: Candy is a firm believer in a natural look, and she sticks to serious hair care and a good diet.
Photo above: Jeffrey Wien.
Photo right: E. Volkovitz, courtesy of Cie.

something new, but don't just do it because it's new and fashionable." Keep an eye on fashion and adapt it to yourself. Try to be unique and always to apply your own personal touch. I know several very interesting women who are unique in their personal style but who never change their hair style; still, they are very much in fashion because their attitudes as well as their clothing are contemporary.

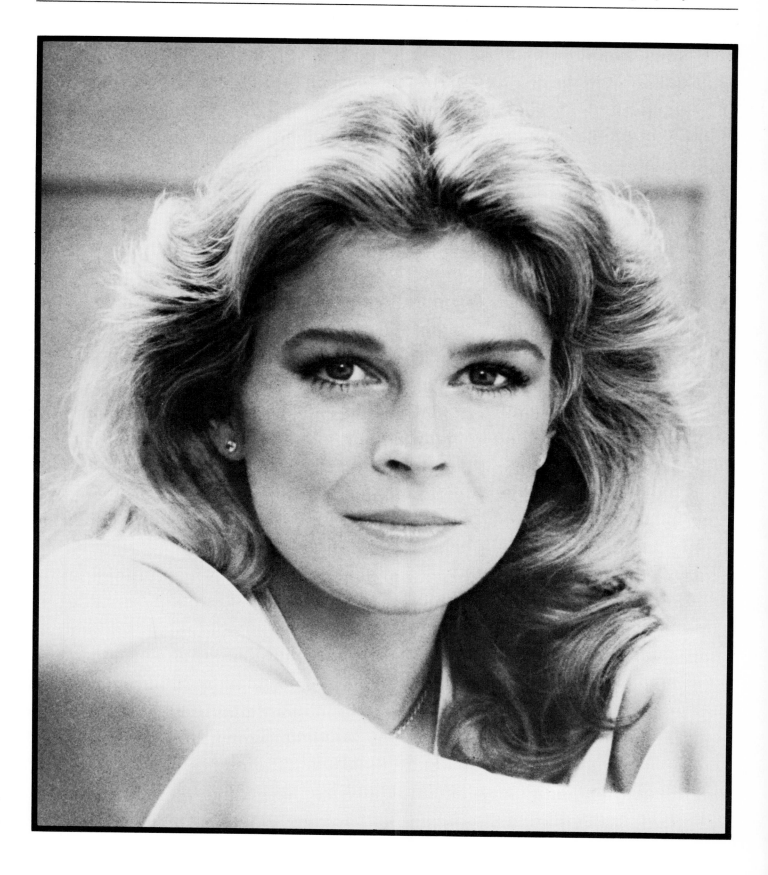

Diana Ross

Diana Ross can handle an extreme or dramatic style because it is consistent with her personality. She prefers to keep her hair long enough to pull back into a chignon and to be able to play it into different styles. Diana is very handy with her hair and uses lots of different techniques. I've learned some good tricks from her.

Gloria Vanderbilt

Black-haired, camellia-skinned Gloria Vanderbilt has fine, straight dark hair, and for this a blunt cut is best. She changes the length within certain limits and turns the ends up or under. The shape of her head and her ears always show, and she has worn her hair this way for at least ten years.

There are a great many lessons to be learned from these unique women. I think it is particularly important to remember not to be a slave to fashion. Try the trends, but always adapt them to *your* look and *your* life, and if you should be lucky enough to find a look that really suits *you,* keep it—*you* may be the one that starts the trends yourself.

The key to finding the "right" hair style for you lies in really understanding your hair. This means taking into account what it will and won't do, the kind of life you lead and the time you have to deal with your hair—and whether you are handy with your hair or not.

As I've emphasized, you must know the real nature of your hair—its texture and degree of curl—before you settle on the look or style that's right for you.

Obviously, the best and easiest kind of style should be one that looks good on you and requires a minimum of upkeep. If you're a busy person and every minute counts, then you probably would like to take the least time to get dressed and put on make-up—say, ten minutes for clothes and five more for make-up. You'd probably like to spend five minutes on your hair (not including washing). For this kind of timing you need hair that's perfectly cut and can be finger-combed or just lightly blown into place with a hand dryer. (For evening you're probably willing to spend a little more time—more about that in Chapter 7.)

But for some women this kind of ease is not so easy to come by, and for others it's impossible. A little more polish, a more definite line or a sleeker look is what you may need to look your best, and this can take more time and effort.

How, then, do you find the "right look," the one that works with the texture and degree of curl that you have and works as well with your life style and requirements?

First, you may have to compromise on the time aspect in the beginning. A hair look that's right for you might require fifteen minutes to execute at first, but you'll find that with practice, the time you spend on your hair will be greatly reduced. Second, you may have to experiment with chemically changing the degree of curl or wave in your hair by perming or straightening.

In addition, you must consider *how you feel* in a particular style. Your hair may be naturally straight as a stick and it may be no trouble at all to take care of, but psychologically you may feel you have more bounce, you look younger and have a brighter attitude with curls. Or the reverse may be true: you have curls and you feel comfortable with something fairly sleek. As I've said, I normally advise a person to go with what she has, but in some cases when a client really feels better with something that's a little more difficult to achieve, we work out something that suits her. In the case of the curly-haired woman who wants a smoother look, I warn her about the cost and possibly drying effects of straightening, and I suggest styles in the curly range. If, after she considers all this and still wants to change to straight hair because it means a great deal to her, I feel she should do it. *She* has to wear her hair and she has to *feel* good about it.

Most long hair can be styled in many different ways. The "right look" for you, as I've said (and maybe too many times!), depends on your hair texture, your degree of curl, the kind of life you lead and the way you feel with a particular look.

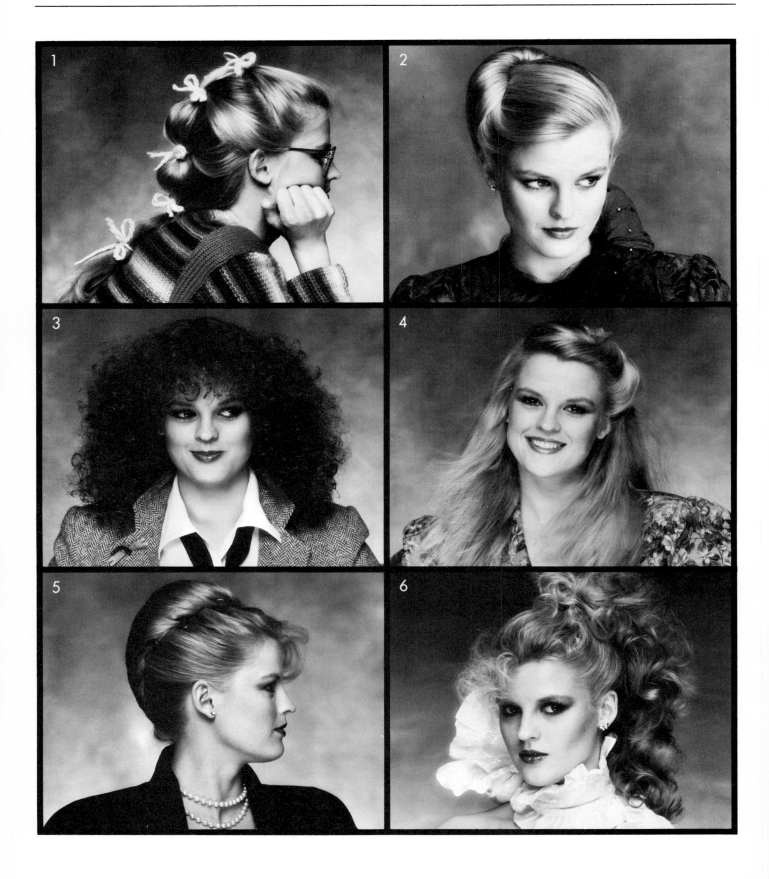

Sara: one face, six different styles Which look is "right" for her?

The pictures on the opposite page show dramatically how you can change your whole look by changing your hair. Each of these styles has a different feeling and gives the impression of a totally different kind of person, yet they were all done on one model, Sara Abrell.

Longer hair gives more opportunity for radical kinds of changes, but short hair also lends itself to different looks (though generally not so different as the ones shown here).

The texture of Sara's hair is medium-fine with soft waves that are not even. Which look is "right" or "best" for her?

The answer, as you can see, is not so simple. First, let's consider what the pictures show. We can immediately see that:

A hair style can radically change your appearance. It can make you look: younger, older, sophisticated, casual, sporty, conservative, trendy. It can be more appropriate for: daytime or evening.

In addition, the *clothes* and the types of *accessories* you wear obviously play a big part in making your hair look one way or another. A French twist (photo 5) can be charming and young-looking with jeans; it can also look serene and sophisticated (and on some women, conservative) with a black crepe dress and classic pearls. The ponytail look (photo 1) is shown with a sweater and tiny wool ties, but it could work beautifully at night with black satin ribbon ties and an evening suit.

As I said above, *time* is another aspect of these hair styles. The very curly look (photo 3) is achieved with a permanent; your hair just needs to be washed and hand-fluffed dry. The headful of soft curls (photo 6) may take a salon visit and a hairdresser's professional skill if you aren't very clever with your hands.

Left: Six different styles on the same model. 1. Ties in a ponytail (see p. 77) 2. Asymmetrical twist (see p. 72) 3. Permanent (see Chapter 12) 4. Partial twist (see p. 72) 5. French twist (see p. 70) 6. Soft-curl setting (see p. 46)

Similarly, the softly twisted sidelock (photo 4) takes less than three minutes to do, while a perfect French twist (photo 5) will definitely take longer.

Which hair look is "right" or "best" for Sara? All of them, in my opinion, look attractive on her. But there are certain styles that work better for her than others.

The look in photo 6 poses several problems. The hair requires setting and skillful combing out; the weight of Sara's hair would make keeping the set for any period of time a problem, and she would probably need to go to a salon to have it done. She would have to make the decision whether she wanted to invest the money and time in visiting a salon to have a hairdresser do it. Also, it is a very special look—more suited for a gala evening and not quite appropriate for an office—so it is not the kind of style Sara could wear comfortably for most of the day.

The asymmetrical twist (photo 2) can be difficult to do perfectly and smoothly if you're not very adept with your hands. It looks lovely on Sara, but she would certainly have to practice a while to perfect this one. This look would be appropriate for an office but is somewhat severe with jeans or sports clothes. It's obviously a very sophisticated look for evening, but do you think it makes Sara look older? I do.

The classic French twist in photo 5 is less "perfect," easier to do by yourself and has the softness of bangs in front. Sara could easily learn to do this by herself. It's a good look with casual clothes and is very sophisticated when worn with evening classics such as pearls and a simple evening suit. She could go to the office with this too.

The soft partial twist (photo 4) is superquick, young and looks pretty with casual clothes and soft dresses. But it could be a problem in an office where "neatness counts" and a young executive look is preferred. This look may not be dressy enough for nighttime.

The knotted ponytail in photo 1 is also young and very charming but takes a bit of work to do. This look with yarn or thin leather ties can go with jeans or sports clothes. With satin ribbons it can look good at night. It's basically a style for when you want to do "something special" with your hair. It's not for the office, in my opinion—too difficult to execute and too fancy.

The curly look in photo 3 is done with a permanent and requires nothing but washing and fluff-drying. The no-time-spent-on-it factor is in its favor, but it may tend to look trendy or faddish and it could be extreme for a rather conservative office atmosphere. This also is a young look and goes well with sports clothes and evening dresses.

I alone cannot totally answer the question as to which look is right for Sara. Only Sara can ultimately tell me which look or looks feel right to her in terms of what she does, where she's going, how she wants to look and the time she's willing to spend to look that way. I can only show her with these styles what she can expect from her hair texture and type, and together we will achieve what is best for her.

Your hairdresser should be able to suggest several different looks for you. You will be helping to guide him by showing photographs of what you want. But ultimately the texture and degree of curl in your hair, the dexterity of your hands and the kind of life you lead will all be decisive factors. You and your hairdresser must work it out together.

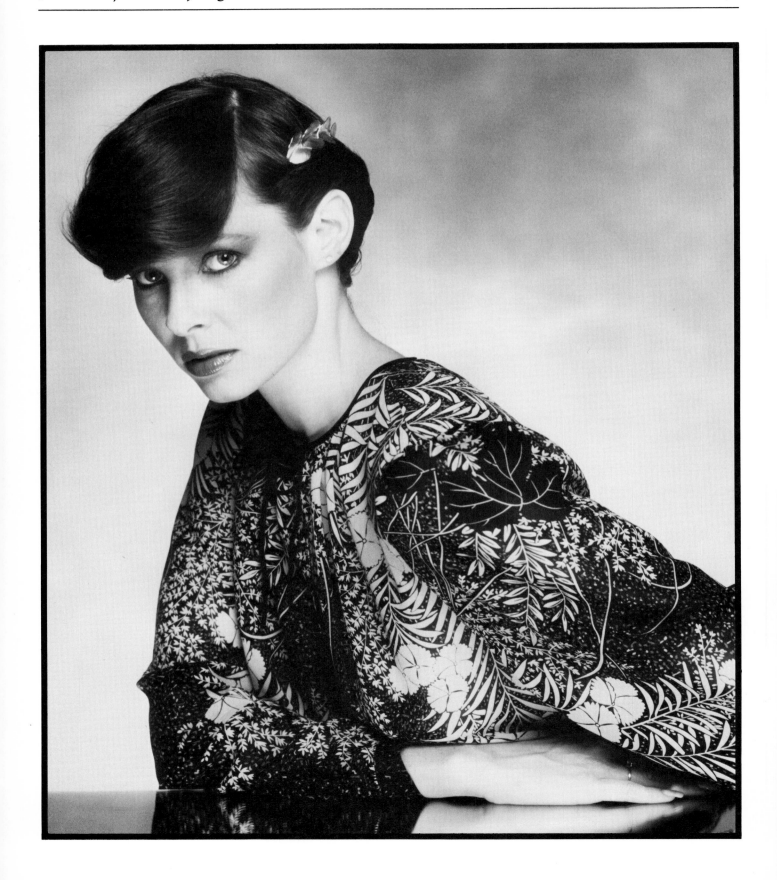

3

Your hairdresser:
finding, keeping, coping

First, you must be able to decide what kind of hair style you like. Look at magazines, look at the people in your office, people on the street, in stores, in movie lines. When you find a hair style you like, go up and ask the person who cut her hair. You'll never know if you don't ask, and most women are flattered if someone tells them their hair looks good and will readily tell you the hairdresser who did it.

After you've found a look that you like in a magazine or a cut that you've seen on someone else, *don't assume that you can have*

Left: Explain the look you like by showing photos from magazines to your stylist.

that cut. A cut or style depends, as I've said before, on the texture and amount of curl in your hair.

Call the salon where the hairdresser is and ask if you can drop by for five minutes for a consultation or make an appointment for a shampoo and set or blow-dry. You want to get a feel for what this person does. You have to feel that his hand is comfortable and knowing. You must sense that this person can cut your hair and you must have a certain confidence in him.

Remember, a famous name or salon does not mean a good cut. It depends on the hairdresser, no matter what or where the salon is.

How to tell a hairdresser what you want

You must be very specific when you are discussing a style with a hairdresser. Some people have different definitions for words. For instance, I find that someone may mean one thing by the word "soft" and I may interpret it as another. So I always ask, "If you can find anything visual, please show it to me." The style in a photograph or magazine article does not have to be exactly what you want. It can be a picture that shows the degree of wave that is right. Find other pictures that define what you want in length, in amount of wave, and for movement and style. I usually ask to see more than one picture because there are so many variables and I want to be sure that I know what the client wants.

The decision on a style really rests somewhere between you and your hairdresser. Some hairdressers think they are gods or artists, so be careful if someone tells you what you absolutely should have. But you yourself are not a haircutter, either, so you must listen, too. It's basically a matter of cooperative effort, and that's why it's so important to be comfortable with a hairdresser. Once the cut is started, give the hairdresser a chance to finish first unless you see grave danger lying ahead and must caution him, but if you've been clear and he's explained what's possible with your type of hair, there should be no disasters.

What if you want to go to another hairdresser in the same salon?

It often happens that you want to try a hairdresser that's in the same salon as the one to whom you are regularly going. In many cases a woman really likes her hairdresser but she doesn't like the style she's getting. Do not hesitate to change hairdressers. It's a bad idea in the long run to stay with someone you don't like, and we usually sense when a woman wants to work with someone else. The best way to make the change is to tell the manager that you like his salon and don't want to leave and that you feel someone else might do better with your hair and could he please arrange it. Managers are usually hired for a sense of diplomacy and tact as well as other factors, so let him work it out with the hairdressers involved.

How do you know if you have a good haircut?

Don't think because the price is high the cut is good, and don't think that the amount of time spent on cutting the hair indicates that either. Haircutting time depends on the individual operator. An equally good haircut can take fifteen minutes or an hour. When I play with hair too long, the form doesn't come out right. I have to work quickly. That's my temperament. One thing I can say, though, is that fast or slow, every section of the hair that's to be cut must be small. I make ten sections where another hairdresser might make two. You cannot skip steps. I just happen to do all the steps very quickly.

After you get a cut you usually leave the salon looking beautiful. The most important question in evaluating if you have had a good cut is how easy it is for you yourself to duplicate the look you have come out of the salon with. By "duplicating the look" I don't mean cutting your own hair; I mean combing, brushing, blow-drying or styling your hair as it was done for you in the salon. It should never take you more than a half-hour to achieve the same effect unless you have really thick, long masses of hair. Please remember, however, that you cannot exactly duplicate the look, because you don't have eyes in the back of your head and your arms simply can't go that far. But you should have a fairly good facsimile of what happened in the salon.

Finally, a haircut should be judged on how manageable it is over a four- to six-week (or longer) period. Once the hair gets longer, the style may change but the cut should still keep its good shape over a period of time, even though that shape may change slightly according to the length of the hair. I have known a cut to keep its shape for up to eight weeks or even longer.

For medium to short hair the cut should look its best by the second, third and fourth week. Between four and six weeks you probably will need another cut.

For long hair (below shoulder-length), you need a cut anywhere from six weeks to every three months. You cut to keep hair in a healthy condition. If you don't cut off the dead ends, your hair cannot keep its shape and health. Don't forget, the hair gets its nutrition from the scalp, and the longer it is, the less help it gets from its roots.

What can you do if you have a disaster of a haircut?

When you cannot handle your hair yourself or if you find a near-bald spot, don't panic and don't condemn the hairdresser yet. Go back to the salon and explain your problem to him. Your hairdresser may decide to recut or tell you to wait a couple of weeks and then he will trim again. If you don't feel satisfied with the response, ask to see the manager, who may agree with your hairdresser. Try not to be too aggressive about it; your hair will grow—it always does. I suggest that you not ask for your money back but that you not pay for a recut when it's time for one. Sometimes people think we are magicians. We aren't, of course. We can create beauty, but we cannot make your hair grow in one day, so please try to be understanding.

Do the haircuts in magazines work in reality?

Many times a beautiful hair style that you see in a fashion magazine hasn't a chance in the world in reality. This is because the hair on the model's head has to look good for only as long as it takes to shoot the picture. In real life your hair has to look good all the time if a haircut is to "work." There are lots of tricks we use in the studio on hair that is fine and long and won't hold a shape. For instance, all the hair can be pushed to the front of the head to give the look of a luxurious mane, while backstage the head is practically bald. And then, we often use fans to give a movement and lift to the hair that it would never have on its own.

How much should you tip and what about Christmas presents?

Tipping has nothing to do with hair styling directly, but it causes many women a great deal of anxiety because they often feel they are giving too much or too little. Tipping is a subject that's difficult to deal with specifically, because it *is* so subjective. Basically I advise that you give what you would like to, but at the same time you should realize that it is not necessary to leave a tip if you're not satisfied. The general guideline to tipping is 15 percent of the amount for a particular service, but as I said, this is in no way a fixed rule. For example, a haircut may cost you $25 and you're delighted with it; you may want to give the hairdresser as much as $5 or you may feel $2 is enough. According to the 15 percent guideline, the amount should be $3.25, but you must judge what you think is right. I do suggest, however, that you stick to even dollar amounts rather than change. Follow the same guidelines for the person who shampoos your hair, but here it's perfectly OK to give change.

If you are a regular customer, you might consider giving a present at Christmas, but this is really a very personal decision. Some hairdressers prefer money or flowers, others something personal. But don't forget that good hairdressers have many customers and there can be much duplication, especially with colognes, soaps and scarfs, so if you want to give any of these items, it's a good idea to buy them at a store where they can be exchanged.

I have never accepted lavish things, but once when someone offered me a week at her Caribbean house I said yes with great pleasure. I have also accepted books, and artwork made by my clients, but I have refused expensive jewelry that costs thousands of dollars. A tasteful flower in a glass has pleased me as much as the most expensive things. Once, on a Christmas morning when I had been working practically around the clock, one client brought me a huge turkey ready for the oven. *That* was something which was gratefully accepted.

who cuts my hair?

When I opened my first shop I wanted to give Japanese hairdressers a chance. I gave auditions in Japan and I hired three people. One of those three, a woman named Kinuko, absorbed my ideas and work beautifully. She's still with me and she's the one who cuts my hair. She also gives me a mild permanent every two to three months so that my coarse, stubborn straight hair literally stays in shape. I used to go to a barber in Greenwich Village when hair was worn shorter, and he was excellent. But as fashion changed, his techniques no longer worked. Then I began to cut my own hair. When I think back I realize it looked hideous, but at the time I was proud of it. But changes like that are what fashion is all about.

HAIRCUTTING IN THE STRANGEST PLACES

I have often cut hair in ladies' rooms in hotels, airports and railroad stations. This is not because I have a strange passion to do so but because when you're on a photo assignment or making a commercial you have to be prepared for anything.

In more usual circumstances, I often give haircuts (and sometimes perms) to friends in their kitchens.

But the most awkward place I ever did a haircut was in a small private plane en route to Vermont. *Vogue* was doing a cover on Princess Grace of Monaco, and while we were up in the air, Richard Avedon, the photographer, said he needed a haircut and wanted to have it done in the back of the plane. I thought this would be the first and last chance that I would have to give a haircut in the most limited amount of cubic space I could imagine, so of course I cut his hair. He did not seem displeased with the results.

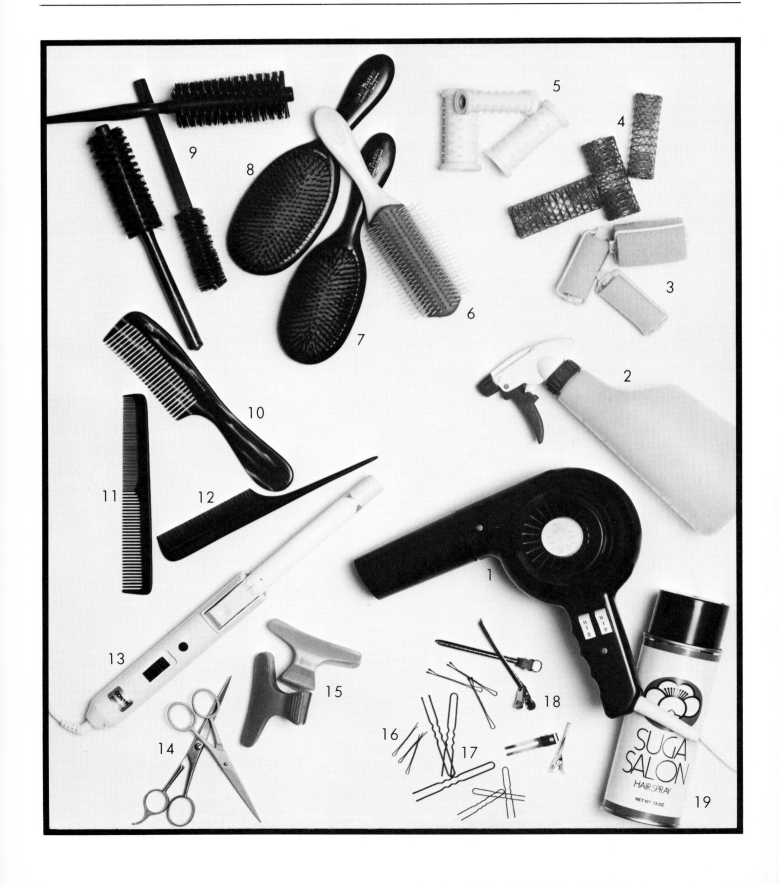

4

The tools the professionals use: what will work best for you

Hand-held hair dryers

In the salon we use hand-held hair dryers for blow-drying and styling. These have high wattage because the more power a dryer has, the faster it dries hair and the sooner the client can be on her way. I use a 1,200-watt hand-held dryer in a basic gun style. For home use you should choose a dryer with about 1,000 watts and

Left: 1. Blow-dryer 2. Mister 3. Sponge rollers 4. Mesh rollers 5. Electric rollers 6. Plastic brush 7. Natural-bristle brush 8. Combination brush 9. Round rolling brush 10. Wet comb 11. Set comb 12. Tail comb 13. Curling iron 14. Scissors 15. Blocking clips 16. Bobby pins 17. Hairpins 18. Long and short clips 19. Hair spray

one that is light enough for you to handle comfortably. One thing I always caution about hand-held dryers: hair doesn't feel heat because it has no nerves, so it can easily be damaged and burned if you hold a dryer on it for any length of time. Keep rotating the dryer so that it never focuses on one section of hair for more than a few seconds.

There are different attachments sold with blow-dryers, but I prefer to use only one. It looks like a plumber's helper and reduces the wind while allowing the heat to dry the hair. The effect you get is of natural air-drying or heat-lamp drying and it takes a fifth of the time.

Brushes

I use primarily four kinds of brushes. The first kind is a brush with widely spaced plastic teeth. The Denman brand is probably the most well-known make for this kind of brush. I use it while styling with a blow-dryer when the hair is wet. I keep using it until the hair is almost dry, and then I finish the look with a combination plastic tooth/bristle brush for medium to coarse hair and a pure bristle brush for fine hair.

The combination brush I just mentioned has widely spaced plastic teeth and short natural bristle tufts which are attached to a rubber air cushion. The brand I have been using for the past ten years is the Mason Pearson brush, and although it is expensive, it is a good investment. It can be used for any hair texture except one that's extremely fine, and it comes in purse size also.

A natural-bristle brush is best for extremely fine and medium hair because it separates the strands and helps to give volume. I use this brush primarily for styling fine hair; it does not work for someone with overly coarse hair because the bristles cannot reach to the roots.

I do not recommend brushing the hair madly for any length of time because it pulls the hair and makes the oil glands of the scalp overly active. The old hundred strokes is a myth I certainly don't believe in. I advise brushing for taking out the tangles and dislodging dust and dirt. If you want to stimulate blood circulation in the scalp, don't brush, but give yourself a good finger massage before or during a shampoo.

A round brush is for blow-dry styling and gives a good bend to the hair. I use three different diameters; the largest is 2½ inches, the second 1½, and the smallest 1 inch. I use any brand that has the right diameter and is natural bristle. The smaller diameters are used for shorter hair and give a smaller curl.

Combs

I use three different kinds of combs. The first is an extremely wide-toothed comb in wood, but plastic will do as well. This is primarily used after shampoos to take out the tangles. The second is called a set comb. It's usually about 7 inches in length; half of its teeth are fairly widely spaced and the other half are spaced closely together. This is really an all-purpose comb and is the most popular one among professionals. I also use a tail comb when I roll hair. Its primary use is to tuck in stray tails or ends of hair, and sometimes I insert it into hair to give it lift and shape.

Scissors

I use 5½-inch-length scissors. I like those made in Solingen or those handmade in Japan. They cost anywhere from $15 to $50. If you are going to trim hair at home, use scissors made especially for haircutting, about 6 inches in length.

My scissors last three or four months and I don't sharpen them, except for handmade ones. I use the same scissors for every type of cut. I don't believe in cutting with thinning shears or razors, and I try always to stick to the 5½-inch scissors because I cut myself with anything longer. However, I have used other kinds of scissors. One day a client called me from the hospital. (Usually I don't make out-of-salon calls, but if someone is sick or very old, of course I'll go.) She told me she just wanted her hair washed and set, but when I got there she wanted a haircut. I had no scissors, but we found a pair of cuticle scissors. Luckily she had very short hair and the cut was fine, even though it took me four times as long to do the job.

Clips

I use only two types of clips, long and short. The long clips hold sections of the hair while I cut, and the short clips are used for pin curls or to hold very small sections of short hair while it's being cut.

Setting lotions

I recommend a nonalcohol base and/or nonsticky, nonflaky kind. Other kinds of setting lotions end up on the clothing and look like flakes of dandruff. Also, some setting lotions coat the hair to excess and the shine is lost. I use the green lotion made by René Furturer for blow-drying, as I find it works best.

Water gun or mister

When hair needs a reset, another blow-dry or just some slight misting to perk up the curl, I use a plastic mister from the five-and-ten-cent store and set it for the finest spray. I use water or setting lotion in it when I am doing a blow-dry or revitalizing a wilting style.

Hot rollers

If not used properly, electric rollers can damage the hair, but not, as is commonly thought, because they are too hot. The damage usually comes from tangling the hair or from anchoring the roller too strongly to the roots, thereby breaking them, or by putting in rollers that are too heavy for fragile hair and thus breaking it. I don't see much difference between the moist and dry kinds of electric rollers. If you wet your hair slightly, you'll get the same effect, i.e., a slightly tighter curl, and you can have control over it by varying the amount of water you use.

Curling irons

I don't normally recommend curling irons for home use, as I have often seen rather severe skin and scalp burns when clients themselves use them. We like to use them at photographic sittings and in the salon because we get quick results and a polished look, but they take a good deal of manual dexterity.

IN HIGH PLACES

Most models are tall and therefore taller than I am. They are usually most cooperative about bending their knees a little so I can do their hair. But one of my favorite models, Veruschka, who is over six feet tall, is the most considerate of all. Whenever I did her hair she always had a box placed next to her so I could stand on it and reach the top of her head.

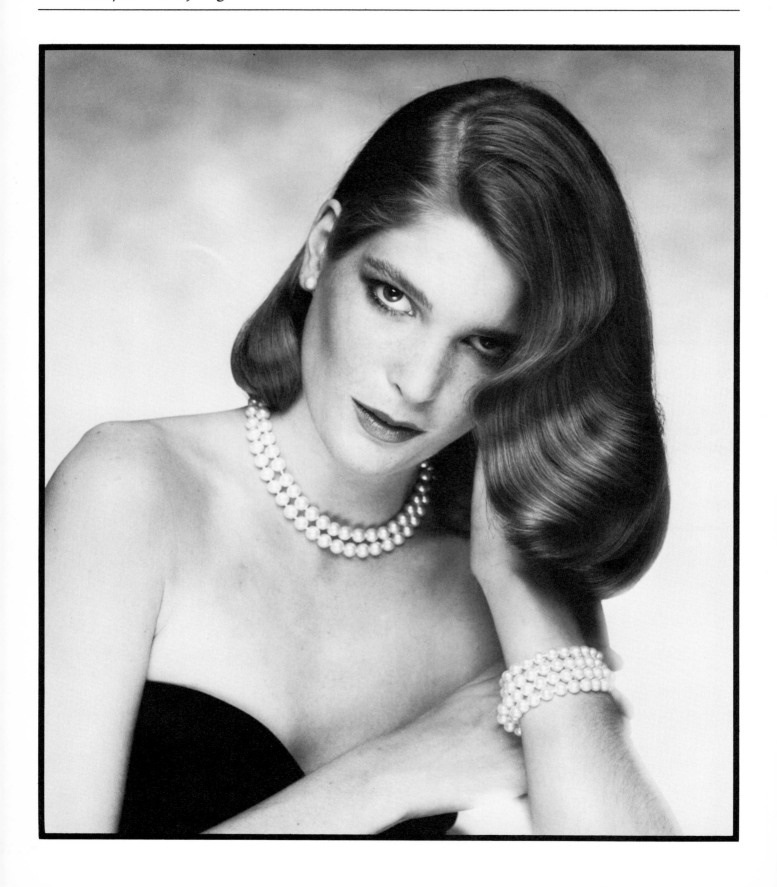

5

What the pros do
with hair setting

Setting means to place or arrange the hair in a certain way. Setting gives the hair definite line and form, based on the way the hair is cut. Some hairdos require setting, others don't. If you've had a permanent, the set has been put into your hair permanently and you probably don't have to do anything more to it than wash, dry and fluff it into place, but if your hair is straight and you want some curl, you will probably choose some method of setting it.

Left: When hair is roller-set, the size of the roller determines the degree of wave. In this style the front is set with 1½-inch-diameter rollers and the rest are 2 inches.

There are many different techniques for setting the hair, and each one gives different results. For instance, one very common method is to wind it onto rollers. Roller setting gives the hair volume, body and curl.

Setting can be done with different implements; you can use bobby pins, hairpins or even old-fashioned kidskin rollers. Braiding the hair is also a form of setting it. You will get wavy, not-so-wavy, curly or not-so-curly effects from each of these different kinds of sets. There is also a special setting technique that we call "wrapping" which makes long hair straight.

You can combine two kinds of settings if you like. For example, when you pin-curl your hair, you may want to put electric or sponge rollers at the crown for extra volume. Or you may want to wrap your hair and just set the bangs. Most hairdressers use all of these techniques to create different hair styles. If you've never tried any of these methods, it's worth your while to experiment and to see what effects you can get on your own. I've listed all the techniques and the results you'll get from each one.

Roller setting

Roller setting was a product of the late fifties and is still a very popular method of setting hair today. Rolling is simply a way of twisting hair onto round rollers in certain patterns. It can be done by almost anyone and the technique is easy to master. Today we often use blow-drying to replace roller setting, but rollers are still useful for certain styles that need lift and body.

The advantage of roller setting is that it gives an even stretch to the hair, thereby making it smooth, and it also gives body. A roller set also shows the shine more easily and gives a certain amount of control over the hair. People who have frizzy hair can get a much smoother texture with rollers, although, of course, the results are temporary. The heat of the overhead or bonnet dryer used with rollers is distributed evenly, so you don't have to worry about overdrying or burning.

The disadvantages in roller setting lie in the time it takes to roll the hair and the time it takes to dry it. There is also the problem of hair separation between the roller sections. I'm sure you've often seen women with smooth long hair, but at the crown the hair separates into definite ridges or sections. There are two ways to avoid this. The first method is this: After your hair is dry and removed from rollers, take a blow-dryer and move it back and forth over the roots. The blow-drying will mix the hair, and the sections or ridges will disappear.

The second way to avoid ridges is to let the hair dry naturally, and then moisten each section except at the roots. Now begin rolling your hair as you normally would and dry under an over-the-head dryer.

If you don't want to run the danger of having crimped hair on the ends, I strongly advise using end papers or setting papers, which you can find at most drugstores. Simply hold a section of hair taut and place the last inch or inch and a half of hair on the setting paper. Fold the setting paper vertically and begin to roll the hair onto a roller (the end paper is rolled first). This takes a bit more time but is well worth the effort because the set will be smooth and the ends won't crimp.

There are several kinds of rollers. Mesh is the most popular because the air goes through the plastic or metal mesh, and drying time is reduced. Plastic rollers are better for people who want to kill frizziness, and sponge rollers will give an extra curl on the ends of the hair and are very easy to handle. I often recommend just moistening the ends of the hair and rolling them on sponge rollers, and in half an hour you'll have a good set without sitting under a dryer.

Do use rollers to maintain the style and line of a cut; for example, two big rollers on top of the crown will give lift, rollers at the nape of the neck can make the hair turn up or under. When you are putting on make-up, use one roller to set your bangs and keep hair off your face.

Warning: A roller set can give you an old-fashioned look if you don't brush it out thoroughly to give it a very natural look.

Hot (electric) rollers

Hot rollers are indispensable to women who want to have or keep a curl or wave in their hair and they want to do it quickly.

The technology of electric rollers changes and improves almost daily. A hair set done with electric rollers does not last as long as one done with pin curls or regular rollers, but you have the major advantage of getting a look in a minimum amount of time. You'll get more curl from a roller with a small diameter (¾ inch) than from one with a larger diameter (1 inch to 1½ inches).

Many people are wary of electric rollers because they feel that they damage and overly dry the hair. The best test for knowing when rollers are safe is that if you can pick up the rollers, you cannot burn the hair. If they are too hot to handle, then wait until they are cool enough to be held easily.

After you have rolled the hair, in-and-out time should be between 3 to 30 minutes, depending on texture and length of the hair. If your hair is fine and fragile and you just want a slight wave, 3 minutes should do it. If you have coarse and healthy hair and you want curls, you can leave rollers in for 30 minutes.

One trick I have to protect the hair from too much heat is to use toilet paper as an end or setting paper. Classy toilet paper is double-layered. Use only one layer and one section, and wrap the

Right: Protect ends from burning and crimping with toilet paper (p. 58). *Opposite:* This style is done with rollers left in the hair for only 3 minutes.

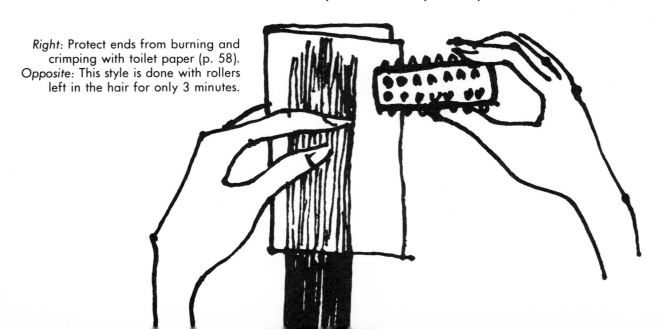

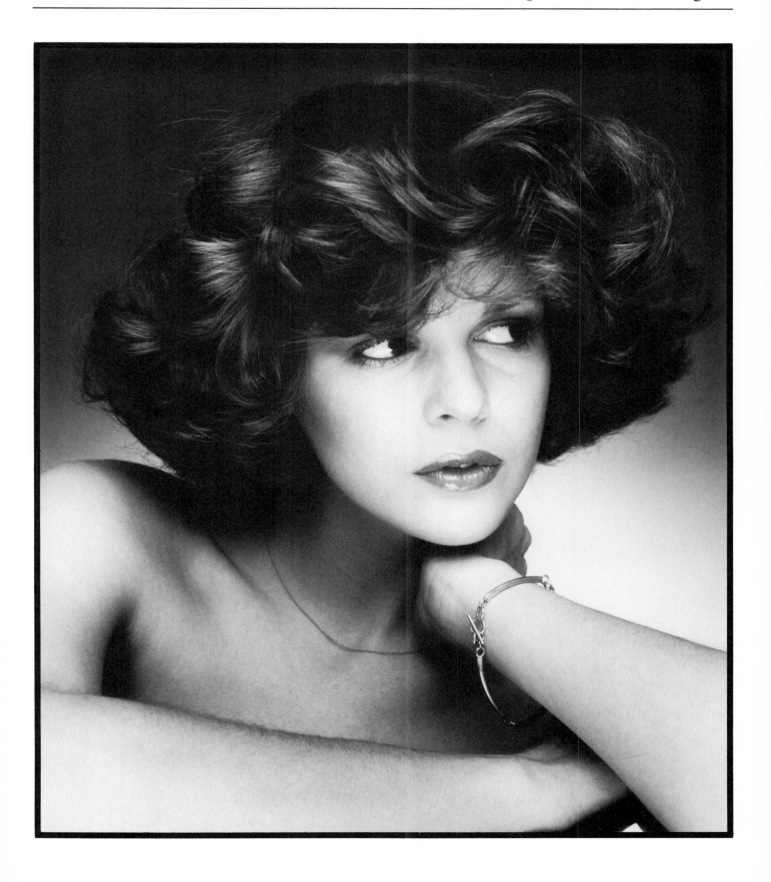

end of the hair with the half of the section, extending the other half above the hair. Start by rolling the empty paper onto the roller; this way the hair will not crimp or tangle or overheat.

For the strongest set with electric rollers, moisten your hand and dampen the ends of hair with your fingers. Then use the toilet-paper wrap and leave the rollers on longer than you normally would. For fine hair, leave them on for 2 to 5 minutes; for undamaged medium to coarse hair, the rollers could stay on for up to 30 to 45 minutes.

If you just want to have a wave or the minimal amount of curl in your bangs, at the crown or at the sides of your head, roll a strand of hair over a curler as you normally would and hold the roller in your hand for 30 seconds to 1 minute. This will give a gentle bend and direction to the hair.

If there is an area of your hair that's being impossible or unmanageable, you can usually tame it by using the hand-held heated roller in that one spot.

When you go to buy electric rollers, look for those with shorter and less sharp spikes and ask how many minutes they will take to heat up. Some brands take up to 15 minutes to heat, and some will be ready to use in 1 minute; obviously I prefer the latter, since no one of us has any extra time these days.

Kidskin rollers

Using kidskin rollers is a very old-fashioned method of setting hair, and you can almost do it with your eyes closed, it's so easy. The effect is similar to that of a pin curl, but the curl is even tighter. This kind of setting gives a young look and works best on long hair. Kidskin curlers are also very inexpensive and can be bought at most five-and-dime stores. A kidskin curler looks like a flattened string bean. These curlers are made of wire about 6 inches long and covered with real leather or kidskin or plastic. Real leather or kidskin is the better kind to buy because they are less slippery than plastic.

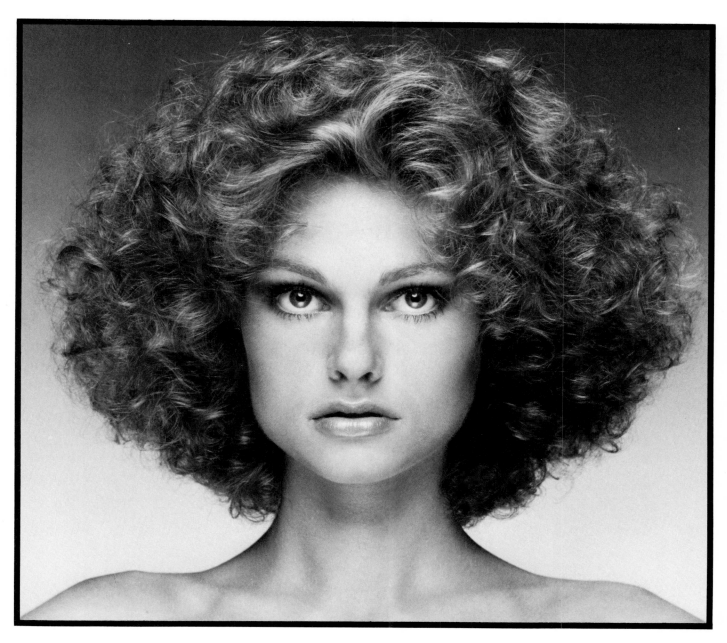

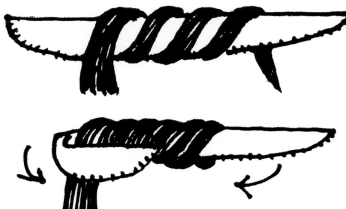

Left: Old-fashioned kidskin rollers are super-easy to use and give your hair the greatest degree of curl and volume *(above).*

The easiest way to use kidskin curlers is to simply roll the hair around the center of the kidskin strip and flatten both ends as if you were wrapping a package. You can also make a U and zigzag the hair around it; the effect is the same as a hairpin curl but with a larger wave. The rows that you set don't have to be straight or perfect, but the amounts of hair in each section should be similar so you get an even amount of curl.

Bobby-pin or pin-curl set

In this type of setting you wind the hair around one or two or three fingers, making it into a flat curl and fastening it with a bobby pin or clips. The more fingers you use, the larger the pin curl will be. You can also go in the other direction and wind hair around a pencil to make very tight or even frizzy curls. A roller set starts with the ends of the hair. Pin curls start at the roots and therefore give a much tighter and rounder curl. Always wind the hair in the direction you want the finished curl to go.

When I want a lot of wave near the roots or when I want to position a wave exactly, I use pin curls. Also, to keep the line or shape of a style (especially a pageboy), I often suggest that you put in a few pin curls at bedtime. And a good time to use a few large pincurls is in the bath when the humidity does its best to

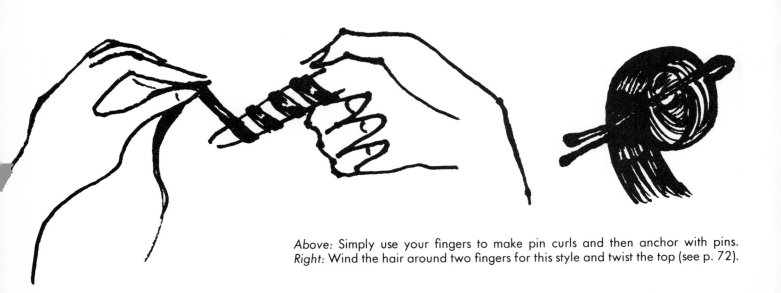

Above: Simply use your fingers to make pin curls and then anchor with pins.
Right: Wind the hair around two fingers for this style and twist the top (see p. 72).

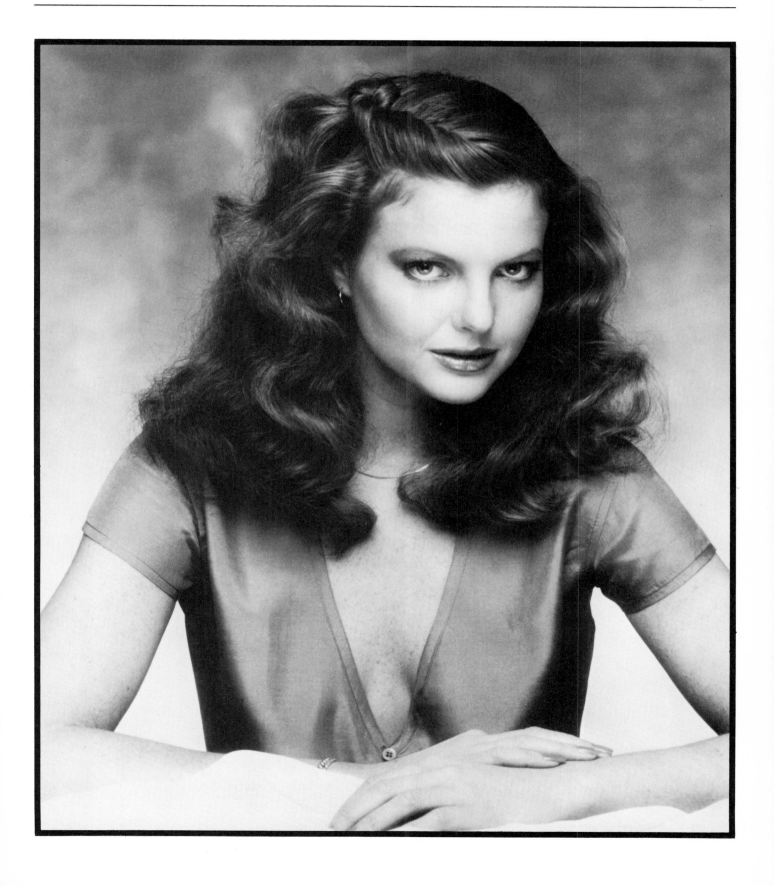

make hair limp or frizzy. You might try tucking a few pin curls under a beach hat so that you can emerge in the evening with your hair looking controlled and polished.

Hairpin set

A hairpin set gives a small wavy zigzag look to the hair, whereas a bobby-pin set makes rounded curls. When you do a hairpin set, don't start with wet hair or it will take forever to dry; just moisten the hair, and using the natural shape of the hairpin, roll the hair around it in a figure-eight shape. Leave the hair to set for one or two hours or sit under a dryer for twenty minutes. Use medium- to large-size hairpins depending on the amount of curl you want. The larger the hairpin, the looser the curl.

Braiding set

The object of braiding hair is to achieve a crimped look when it is brushed or combed out. Divide the wet or damp hair into sections as small as you wish. (The wetter your hair, the more crimped it will become.) The sections do not have to go in geometric rows, nor do they have to be scientifically neat. You can braid your whole head or make specific areas more interesting by braiding them wet and then combing out the braid. Try a small braid on each side of the head or start one half or one third the way down the hair shaft, and braid from there to the end. Braiding will also give a great deal of volume if you do a great many small braids and then thoroughly brush them out with a bristle brush.

Curling irons

I don't recommend curling irons for fragile hair. Even if your hair is healthy and can take a good deal of heat, keep the time spent with a curling iron to a minimum and try to use only one that is coated with Teflon. To achieve the tightest amount of curl,

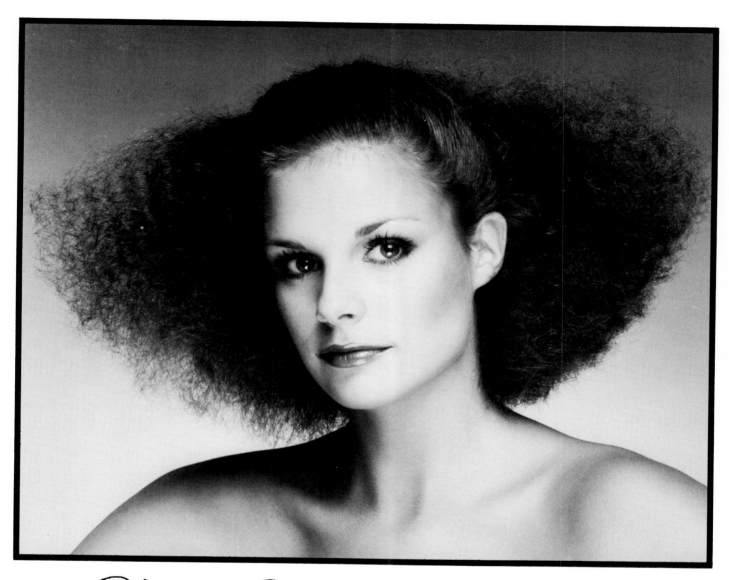

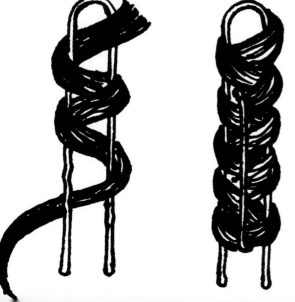

Above: Hairpin sets give wavy zigzag look to your hair. *Left:* Wind hair in figure-8 motion around hairpin and anchor ends with bobby pin up the middle.

use a curling iron on very small sections of hair. Always test a curling iron with tissue paper. If the paper turns color at all, the iron is too hot. Curling irons also require a good deal of dexterity in use because of the danger of the heat, the possibility of burning hair and scalp, and the difficulty in managing them efficiently. I generally advise against them for home use.

Wrapping

Wrapping is a technique that can be put to good use by someone who has very curly or frizzy hair and wants to make it temporarily straight. The hair must be soaking wet to wrap it. If, in addition, you use setting lotion, the results will be even straighter. Start at either the temple or behind the ear and swoop the hair in one direction and then use long clips or tape to anchor it. If you are using an over-the-head dryer you don't need to use a net; with any other kind of dryer, use a good sturdy net to cover the hair. After 20 minutes or more, depending on length and thickness of hair, re-wrap the hair, going in the opposite direction. This technique is very simple and really does straighten the hair, but it has the major disadvantage that it takes almost forever to dry, especially if the hair is coarse and heavy. You can get almost the same effect by setting hair on large rollers and blowing it dry to straightness.

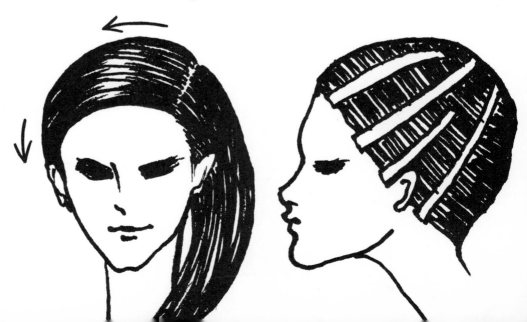

PERFECT PLACEMENT
Once, on a shooting with Hiro, the photographer, on a
Caribbean island, we were in such a remote area that there
was no electricity for rollers, a dryer or a curling iron. After
dinner and way past midnight I finally persuaded the
model, who was with her boyfriend, to sleep with pin curls
all over her head, and it seemed to take hours to do the set.

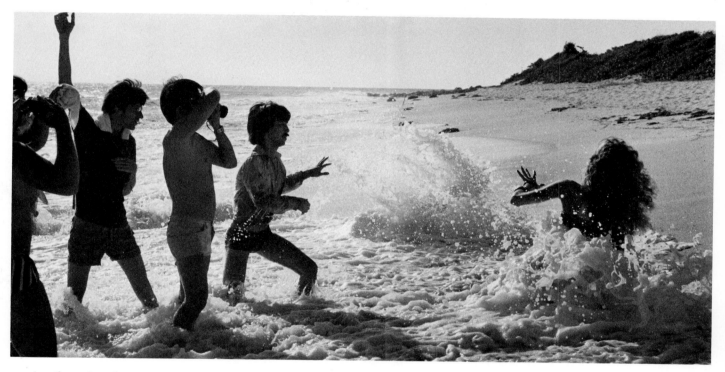

At five in the morning Hiro decided we were going to
photograph on the beach. I told him to please get the shot as
quickly as possible, since the humidity would straighten out
the set in less than five minutes.

Hiro started shooting, slowly backing into the water.
Finally he had the model, who was wearing a charming
white dress, kneeling, and suddenly a huge wave washed
over her. Hiro kept shooting, the hair was of course a
disaster, but back in New York when the art director saw
the shot he thought it was beautiful. In our business, perfectly coiffed hair and perfectly pressed dresses mean nothing—it's the perfect picture that counts.

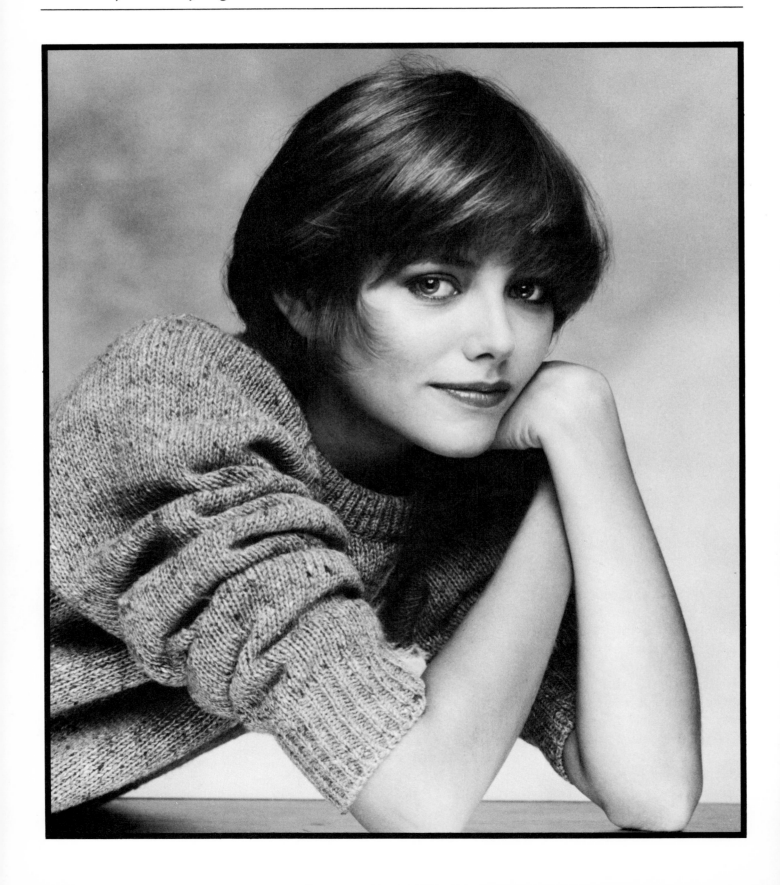

6

All about blow-drying

Blow-drying is probably the most common method of doing hair today. It's a technique that requires some practice, since you must learn to use your hands and a dryer and brush. I start blow-drying hair by using my hands and the dryer. Then, after the hair is about 50 to 75 percent dry, I work with a brush and dryer together.

If you have short hair, start by fluffing or lifting hair away from the scalp with your fingers, keeping the dryer moving lightly over the area where your fingers are working. This fluffing action gives the hair volume. When the hair is about 75 percent dry,

Left: If your hair is this short, just use your fingers and the dryer to ''set'' the look.

start using a brush to give it the line you want: the wide-set plastic-tooth brush made by Denman is ideal for this next process. After you have fluffed, run the brush through your hair to take out the tangles.

Now begin to outline the way you want your hair to fall by catching it in the Denman brush in the *opposite* direction from which you want it to go, then rolling it lightly in the direction you want the hair to fall. Keep repeating this motion over and over, making sure that you don't hold the dryer over any part of the hair for more than a second or two. You can start from the bottom or the sides and finish at the crown, but with short hair the crucial factor is not where you begin blowing but that you keep the brush and the dryer moving constantly.

If you want a curlier look, you need to use a round bristle brush after you have used the Denman brush. The smaller the diameter of the brush (they come in several sizes), the curlier the final outcome will be. For very short hair I recommend the 1-inch-diameter brush.

After you have fluffed and then worked with the Denman brush, you can begin to use the round brush—your hair should be almost dry. Start at the bottom layers of your hair and proceed to the sides and crown. Section your hair horizontally in 1-inch to 1½-inch layers (you don't have to be exact), and roll the hair in each layer over the round brush as you would for a roller set. Move the dryer over each section for three to five seconds, let that section cool for two to four seconds, and then quickly but gently pull the brush out of the hair after each roll. Make sure you release the brush quickly, otherwise your hair will start to straighten out. Keep rolling and drying until you finish your whole head. Shake your head from left to right a couple of times; then run a Denman brush lightly over the outer hair to smooth it, if you like.

If your hair is medium to long, start with fluff-drying it with your fingers and a dryer. After a couple of minutes, bend over, head pointing toward floor, and continue fluff-drying until about 50 percent dry. By holding your head down and hand-fluffing in this way, you will begin to get volume to the hair.

Now stand up and start sectioning it horizontally from the nape of the neck in 1-inch to 1½-inch sections, and begin to use a round bristle brush (with a 1½-inch to 2-inch diameter). Roll the hair gently around the brush, holding the dryer over each section for a second or two. The bottom section is crucial because it is the foundation for the rest of the hair, so be especially careful here. Work up from the nape of the neck to the crown in the back, then begin on the sides, making sure your hair is symmetrical on each side. Save the crown for last.

Start sectioning the crown, working from the back to the front. Pick up the hair on the brush in the *opposite* direction you want the hair to fall and then roll the hair over the brush in the direction you do want it to fall. This scooping and rolling motion gives the hair volume and raises it from the roots. If you want even more volume, hold the dryer over the brush for two to four seconds, let that section cool for three to five seconds, and then release the hair gently from the brush. After finishing with the round brush, mix hair together to avoid sections or ridges, by using the Denman brush lightly all over the head.

For a stronger "set," use a lotion labeled for "blow-drying." Anything else will tangle and mat it.

Please, hold the dryer no closer than 2 inches from the hair; otherwise the heat will damage it. Don't ever hold the dryer in one spot for more than four to five seconds.

Special tips for short hair

While your hair is damp, put some pin curls around the face and at the sideburns. This gives direction to the hair and makes it lie flat, and sideburns always look unattractive unless they are lying close to the cheekbones. If you want to have more volume at the crown, use two or three small sponge rollers (½ inch to ¾ inch in diameter) on the crown while you are blow-drying other sections. Lightly run dryer over rollers until hair is dry, remove the rollers and mix your hair lightly with a Denman brush.

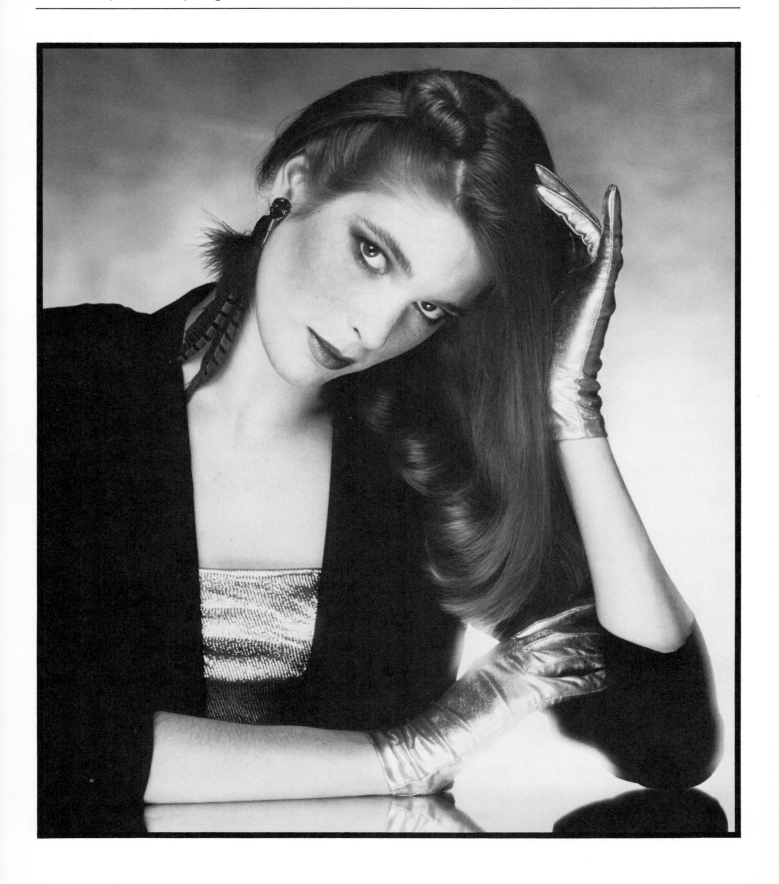

7

Short, medium or long:
salon techniques
you can use yourself

There are many new as well as traditional methods for achieving different looks with hair. Each of the techniques we use in the salon—for example, finger combing, finger waving, twisting, tying, braiding, etc.—gives a different effect to the hair. Some techniques can only be used with long hair, while others are better for short or medium-length hair. In order to give you some guidelines about which methods will work with your hair,

Left: This kind of knotting is easily learned, can be done fairly quickly and gives a very glamorous feeling to most longer hair styles. For "how-to," see p. 79.

I've divided them according to those that will work for "Short to Medium-Length Hair" and those that are more practicable for "Medium to Long Hair." Try some of the techniques that you aren't familiar with or that you haven't used before. Many of the things I've described here are ways we deal with hair for the fashion magazines. Give yourself a little time to experiment; some methods may be a little tricky to execute if you have not had practice, and remember, often, just by doing something different to your hair, you may discover a look or a style that's just right for you.

For short to medium-length hair

Finger combing

Finger combing works best on short-layered wavy or curly hair and gives it volume and shape. After shampooing, towel-dry your hair thoroughly. Now use your fingers as you would a hairbrush, and give the hair lift and line by running your fingers through your hair in a brushlike movement. Repeat the brushing and lifting motions until your hair is almost totally dry. At this point, start brushing with a plastic Denman brush or comb to give a final polish to the style. Continue brushing until completely dry. This should take no longer than a minute. If you want extra body, lightly spray setting lotion (not the sticky kind) on your hair after towel-drying and proceed as above.

If you want to revive a wilting hair style and you don't have time to shampoo your hair, spray it with a fine mist of water and finger-comb until dry. Note: This trick won't work if you have oily scalp or hair.

Right: Finger combing is simple, takes very little time and works best on short, layered wavy or curly hair to give it volume and shape—a perfect technique for traveling.

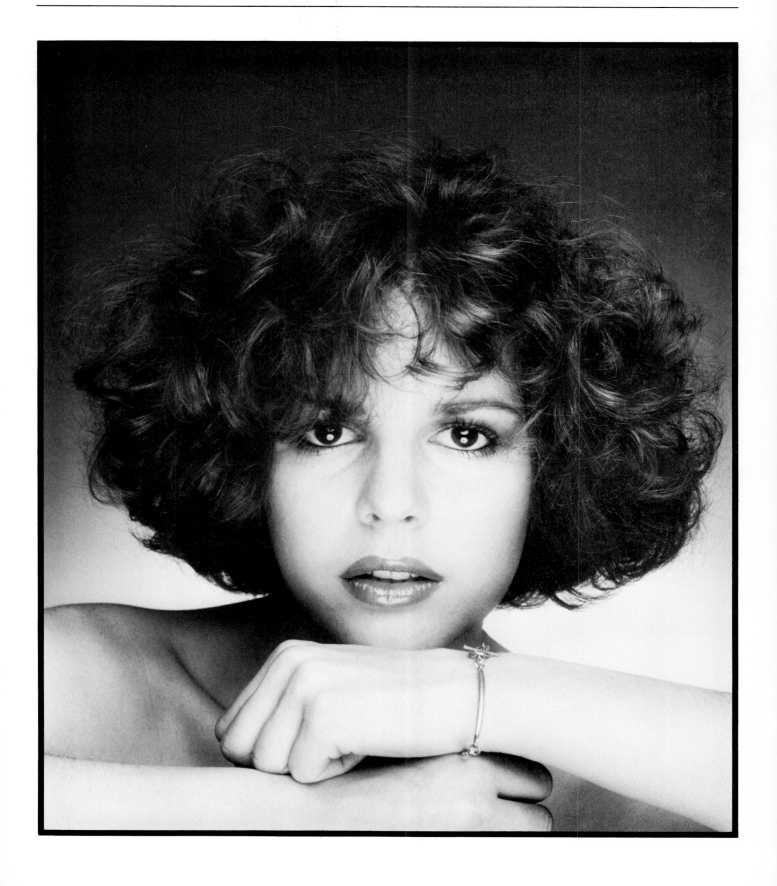

Finger waving and placing

This kind of style/set works best on naturally curly or wavy hair or hair that has a light body permanent. Shampoo your hair and use a setting lotion if you want more body. Towel-dry lightly. Use a wide-tooth plastic brush or comb and shape your hair into its natural wave line. Use clips and tapes to keep the hair flat and the waves in place. Don't touch the hair until it is completely air-dried naturally or has been under a heat lamp or over-the-head dryer. The finished look can be brushed out with a wide-tooth plastic brush or the hair can simply be left in place without brushing for a more "finished" kind of look. Don't use a bristle brush on this because it will mix the hair too much and will loose the sharp definition of the wave line.

Taping

This method works for really short hair and for taming hairs around the face and neckline. Taping makes the hair lie flat or gives it a slight curve or curl. To make hair lie flat, just comb it into place and apply the tape where the hair is likely to pop up. To make the hair bend or curve also, comb it into place and place the tape where the bend or curve is. I prefer to use the pink tape that's labeled "Especially for Hair Setting" (you can find it in most drugstores) or if you don't have that on hand, use Scotch Magic Tape. The tape should remain in place until the hair is completely dry. Here's a good tip: Use the tape when you are taking a bath and don't want the humidity to ruin the line of your hair style.

Right: Use tape to flatten any area of your hair, especially at the nape of the neck or bangs. Special hairdressing tape is made for painless removal.

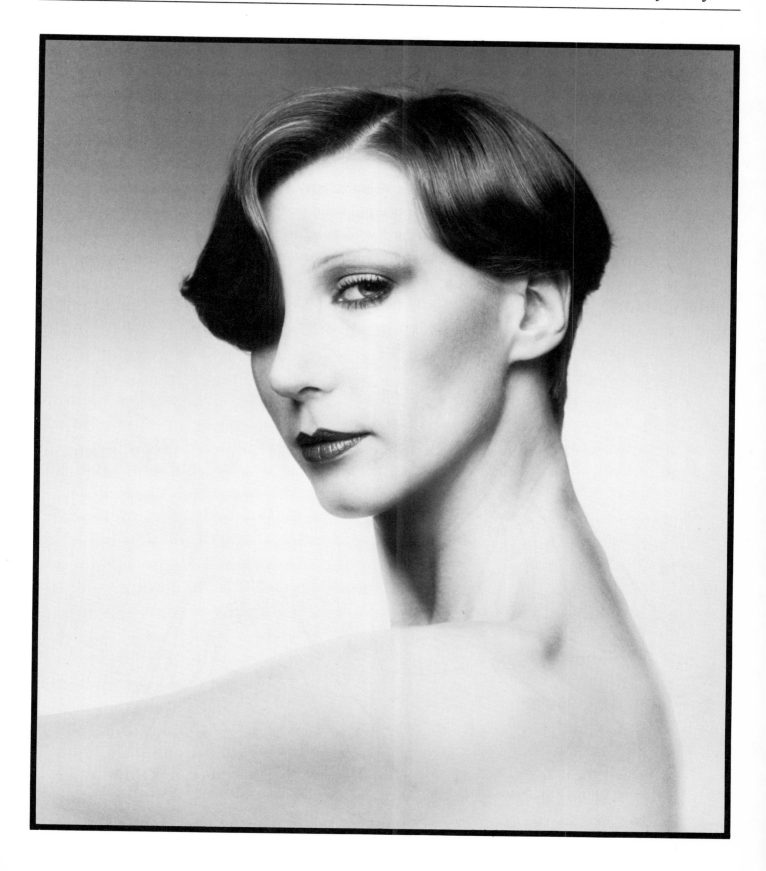

Brush-drying

This technique works best on straightish hair, gives lift and line, and can also be used in a pinch when you're traveling and you've left your hand dryer at home.

After shampooing, towel-dry your hair thoroughly. Using a natural-bristle brush with wide plastic teeth (see page 38 for illustration), begin to make a circular motion with your brush and hands, brushing and patting or rolling your hair into place. Keep brushing your hair in a circular motion all over your head, first with your chin down and then with your head back. Standing is the best way to get the right motion here. If you want an extra bend or curl after finishing, put in a few pin curls or roll the hair on sponge rollers, leaving it for fifteen minutes until completely dry.

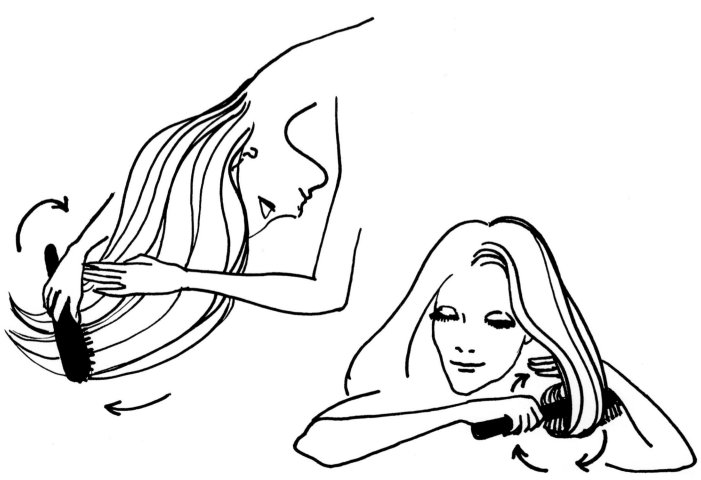

Teasing or back-combing

Most of us are familiar with this technique of fluffing the hair and giving it height by recombing it from the roots. Teasing gives volume and mixes the hair, but there are two *don'ts* that I strongly advise you to heed:

Don't think in terms of bouffant or bubble hair styles and tease hair all over the head. This is an old-fashioned and unnatural look, where the hair has no movement at all.

Don't use spray and tease at the same time; the hair can move even less, and most often it ends up looking like a battered sculpture.

Teasing does have its uses in contemporary hair styles. It can give volume and lift at the crown or it can be done gently before hand-rolling the hair to give it volume and a full line. The best and only way to back-comb or tease the hair is to do it *gently*. Holding the hair taut and in the opposite direction from which you want it to lie, begin, about 2 to 3 inches from the roots, to push the comb gently toward the scalp. Do this pushing two or three times only and do it gently, and then go on to the next section. After you have finished, use a natural-bristle brush to shape the hairs over the back-combing to give it a natural look.

Rough or constant back-combing does contribute to hair breakage and damage because you are going against the hair shaft when you comb or push the hair down, so please use it as little as possible and with as light a touch as you can.

Photo, courtesy of *Vogue*, Condé Nast Publications, Inc. Photographer: Avedon

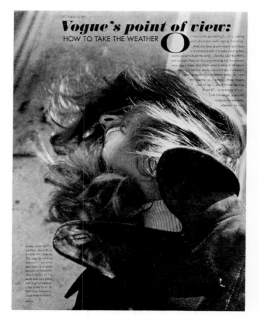

THE QUICKEST HAIR STYLE EVER

The quickest hair style I have ever done was to brush the model's hair and place two huge fans next to her to make her hair move as if it had never been set.

For medium to long hair

Twisting

Twisting gives a beautiful, feminine and finished look to the hair. The best-known kind of twist is the French twist, which has long been a favorite style of women who want a classic, sophisticated look. A perfect French twist is rather difficult to execute. When done in the salon, it can look perfect because, of course, the hairdresser can work with the back of your head. But there are some professional tricks that you can do at home to give yourself a very sleek look.

If you are right-handed (if you are left-handed, reverse the directions), push all the hair with your left hand to the right of your head, then anchor the hair with bobby pins in a pattern that resembles cross-stitch sewing. (The crucial point is to make a firm bobby-pinned base under the hair to be twisted.) Then, with a brush, twist the hair on the right over the bobby pins, twisting in an upward manner with your chin up—otherwise the hair will loosen. After it is twisted into place, anchor it with a hairpin at the crown. Now both hands are free.

Below, opposite: Make a firm bobby-pinned base under hair to be twisted.

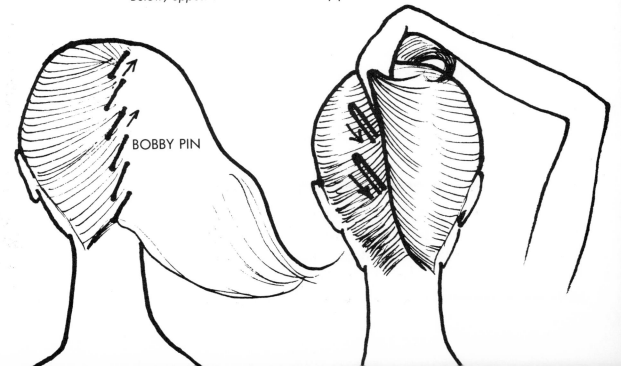

BOBBY PIN

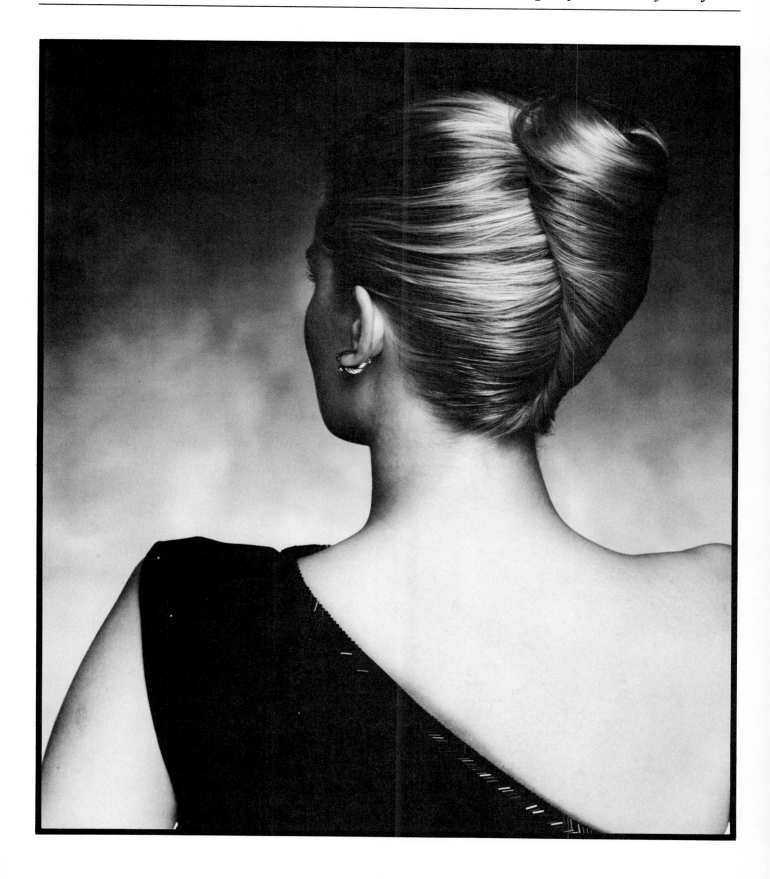

Hold the roll with your left hand and place hairpins (or bobby pins) in the direction according to the drawing. *Important:* The pins must be placed in the opposite direction from which the hair is twisted.

You can do a French twist with wet hair or you can use oil or hair conditioner on the hair. The last two are good ways to keep hair in condition while you're under the hot sun or on a beach. The oiled effect is sleek as a seal, trim and very sophisticated, and at the same time your hair suffers no damage from the sun because it is protected.

French twists do not have to be placed only in the back of your head. They can be done asymmetrically behind the ear or along the top of the head.

Partial twisting

This kind of twisting is used mostly to keep the hair off the face. Simply twist your hair as you would a piece of fabric—the hair should be wet or moist. To me, the prettiest twist is when the hair from the temple to the ear is twisted up and to the back. Twists must be securely anchored, or they roll out easily.

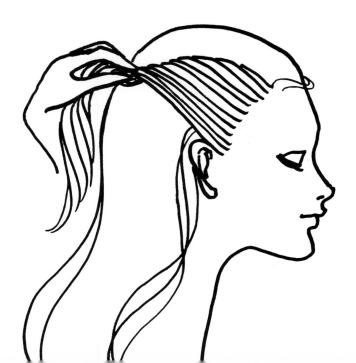

Opposite: Partial twisting is quite easy to do and gives your hair a very finished look. *Right:* Take as much hair as you want in the area from temple to ear, moisten, hold taut, and begin to twist as you would twist fabric. Anchor behind ear with bobby pin or flower.

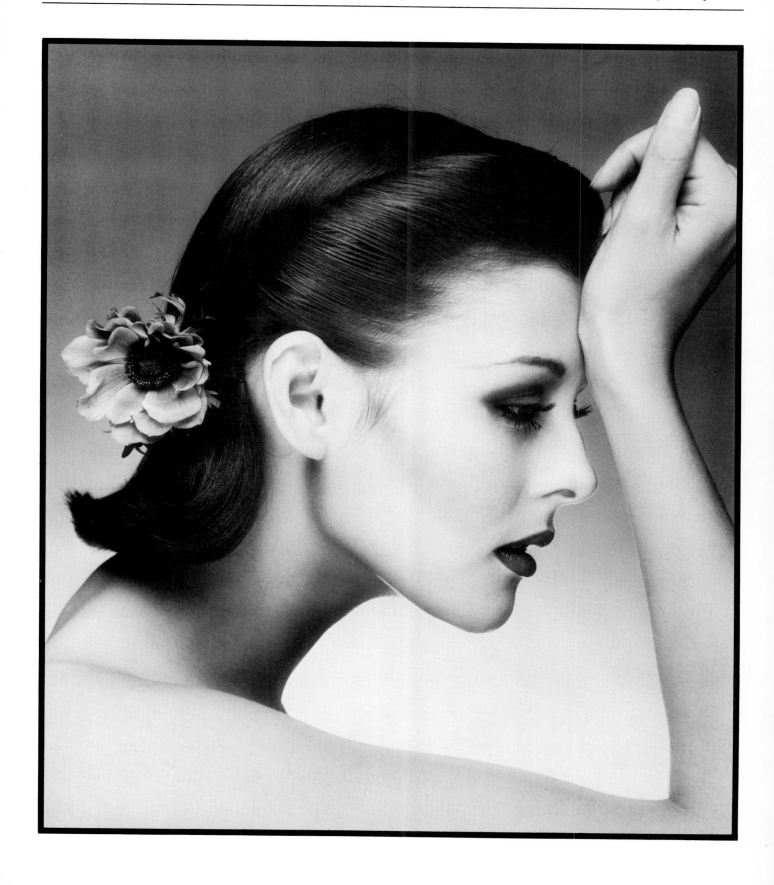

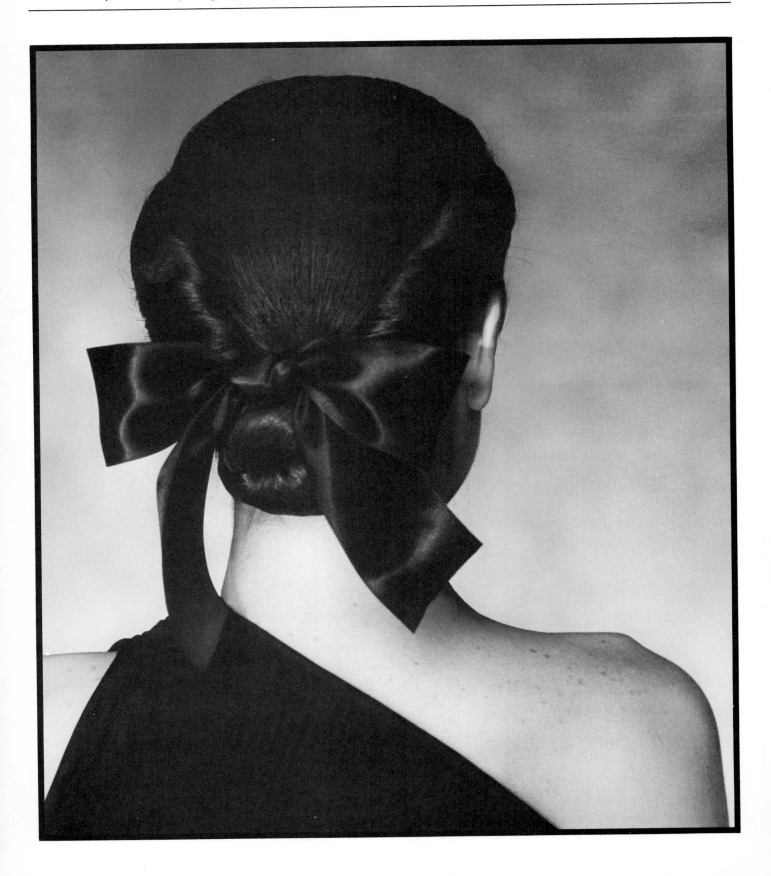

If you are doing a twist on either side of your head and your hair is just long enough, you can connect the twists to each other with ribbons or strings, barrettes or pins or even jewels. Or the twists can be turned into chignons. Don't worry if your twists are not perfect; it's charming to find a woman who cares enough about her hair to give it an extra little fillip, and imperfection here only adds to a pretty look.

Tying

Tying the hair means simply taking strands or sections of hair and tying a ribbon or thread or whatever you want around them. You can really have fun with this. Let your imagination run free and use color as you wish. Try strings, wool, thin suede leather straps, silk cords; the choice of ties is dictated by whether you want a more or less formal look. Ribbons are charming for a younger girl and very romantic. Leather is quite sporty, especially with blue jeans. I have used needlepoint thread and have mixed many colors together. Gold and silver threads are best for evening looks. You might try keeping a collection of strings and ribbons from the wrappings of Christmas presents—they can inspire interesting hair ideas.

You can tie small sections or large sections of the hair. The key is to make sure you knot the ribbon or yarn, etc., securely. To do this you simply make a square knot and cut off the ends very short or let them hang to the length that suits you. If the thread is slippery, tie a double knot. If your hair is wet, you have more control over the smoothness of the look, but remember that when your hair dries and you take out the ties, you'll have ridges.

Left: This style combines a twist and a chignon and is a very sophisticated look. Use the invisible-hair-net trick described on p. 117 to give the smoothest line.

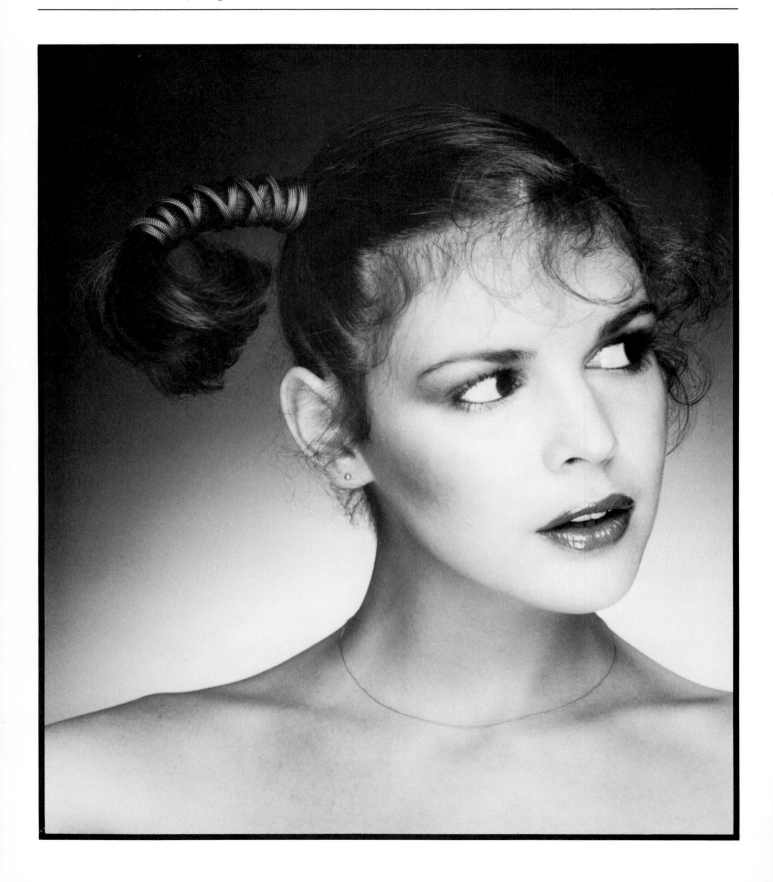

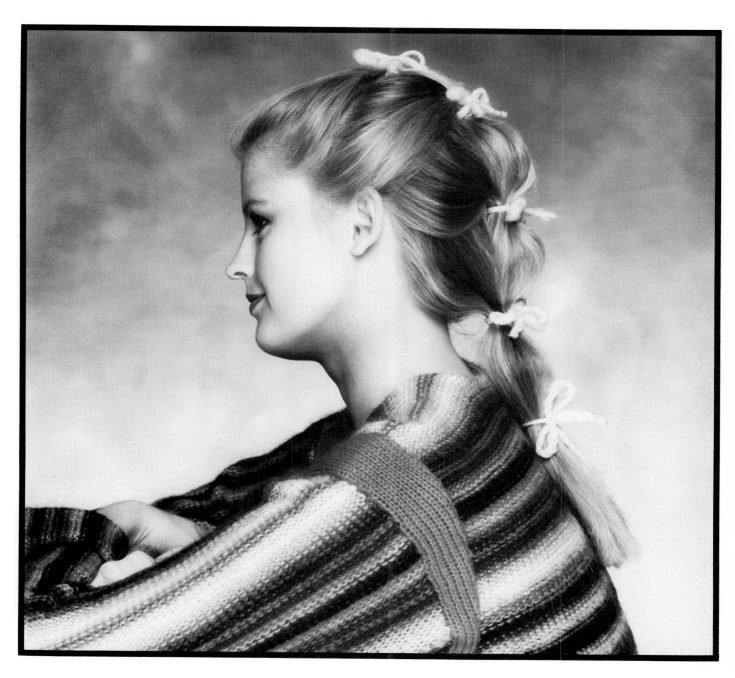

Left: This ponytail is placed in an unusual spot and the hair is left in soft wisps around the face. Anchor the tail with a coated elastic band at the base and then wrap or tie it with colored silk cords that you can find in a notions shop.

Above: Tying can be sporty or dressy, depending on the type of thing you use to tie the hair with. Here, wool yarn is used to tie a ponytail, and the resulting look is very casual.

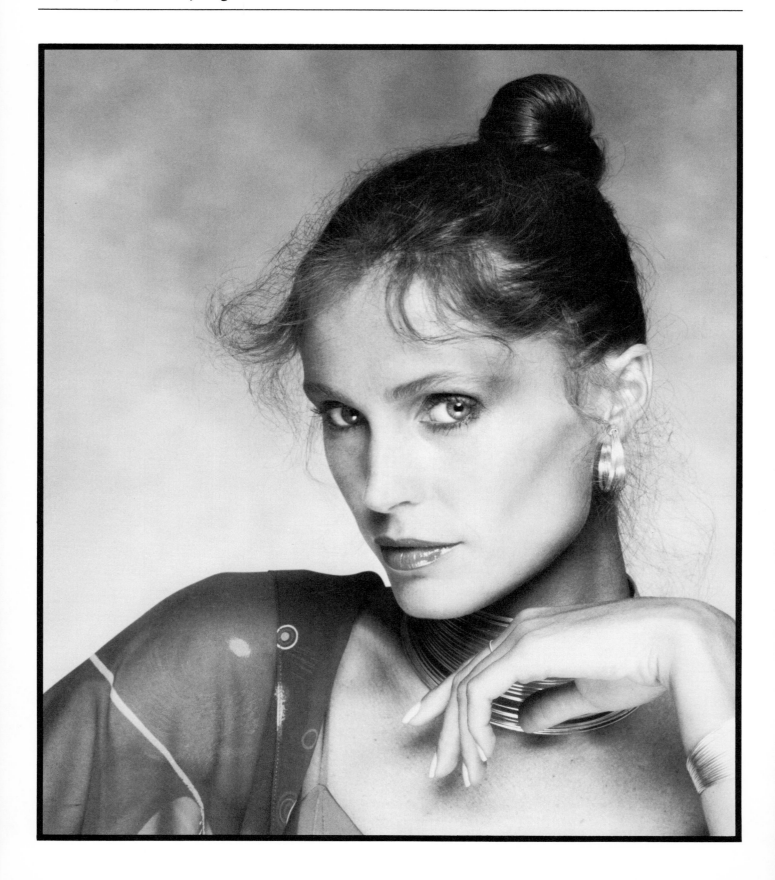

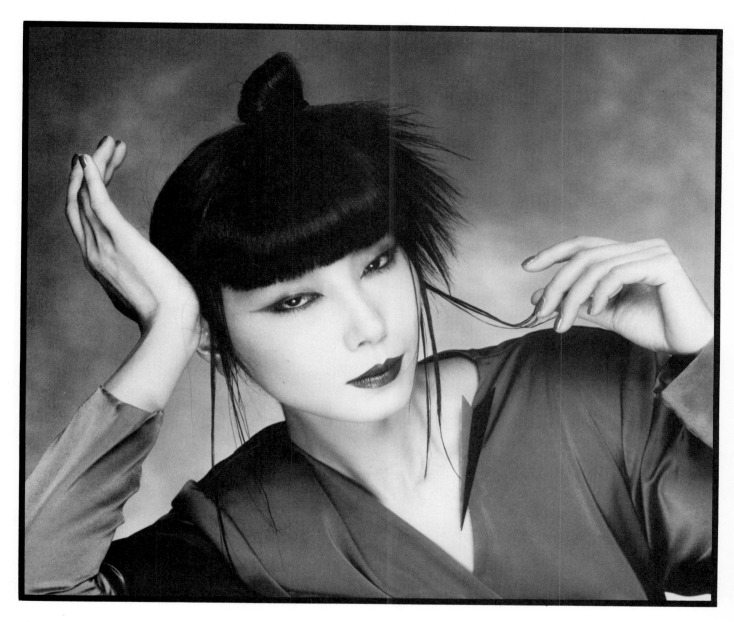

Above, left: Little topknots are quick and easy to do. They're perfect for almost any hair type from straight to naturally curly and they can even look good on hair that's not quite clean.

Knotting

The most common form of knotting is a chignon which comes in either a doughnut or figure-eight shape. Usually chignons are at the nape of the neck, but they can also be done as top knots or front or side knots.

To make a neat, pretty top knot, brush all the hair into one hand, making a ponytail at the crown of your head. Before you anchor it, spray either water or lotion onto a cotton ball and smooth the hair flat all over the head so there are no frizzies or ends standing up. Then take a coated elastic band and wrap it as tightly as you can at the base of the ponytail. Now brush the loose hair thoroughly, and moisten your hands with water, lotion or conditioner and twist it. If your hair is long, twist it tightly to about 4 or 5 inches from its base; if shorter, twist as much as you can. Then, holding it at the end farthest away from the scalp, push it like a plunger into the elastic-band area and it will automatically loosen and give a pretty, soft, round knot. Twist the ends of the hair around and under this looser knot, and use bobby pins or hairpins to anchor. When the hair is thick, use large hairpins. You can place this kind of knot at the nape of your neck or on the side or at your ear.

Rolling

In some ways rolling looks similar to twisting, but usually the rolled hair looks plumper and rounder than twisted hair. I like to roll hair from the front of the face to the back of the head because it's more flattering around the face and neckline, and I like the crown fairly flat so that it shows the shape of the head. If

Opposite: It takes a little time to master the art of rolling, but once you have it the results are well worth the effort.
Right: Start rolling hair in segments from the front and pin into place. Continue until you reach the nape of the neck, then pin ends under the roll. More details on p. 84.

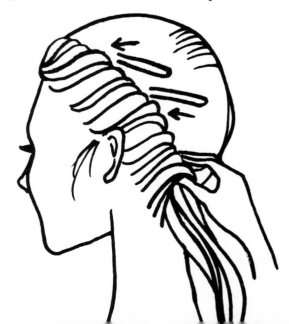

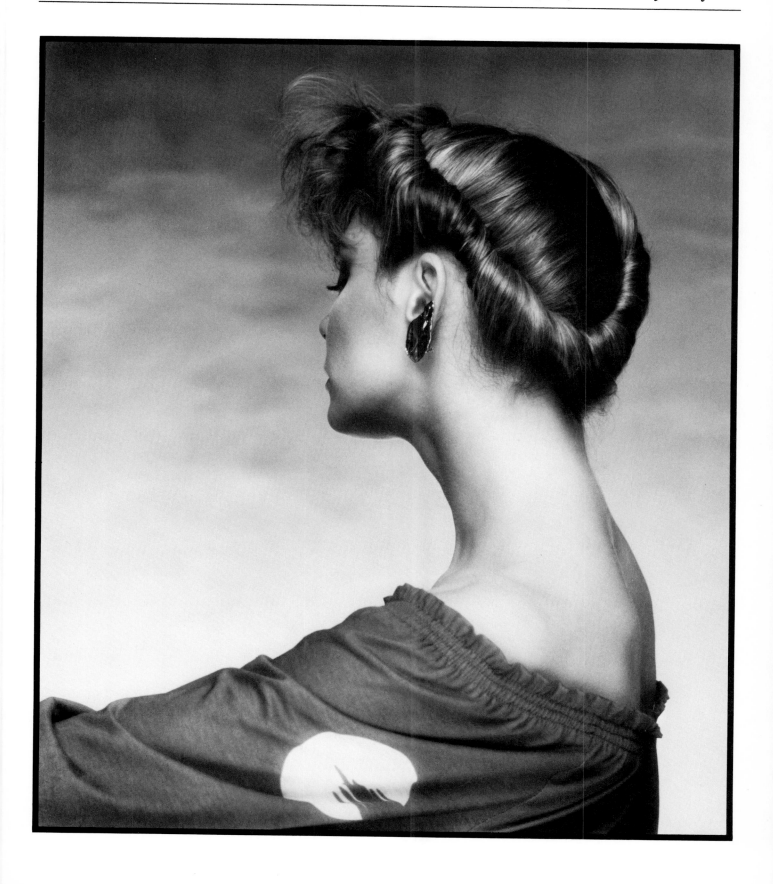

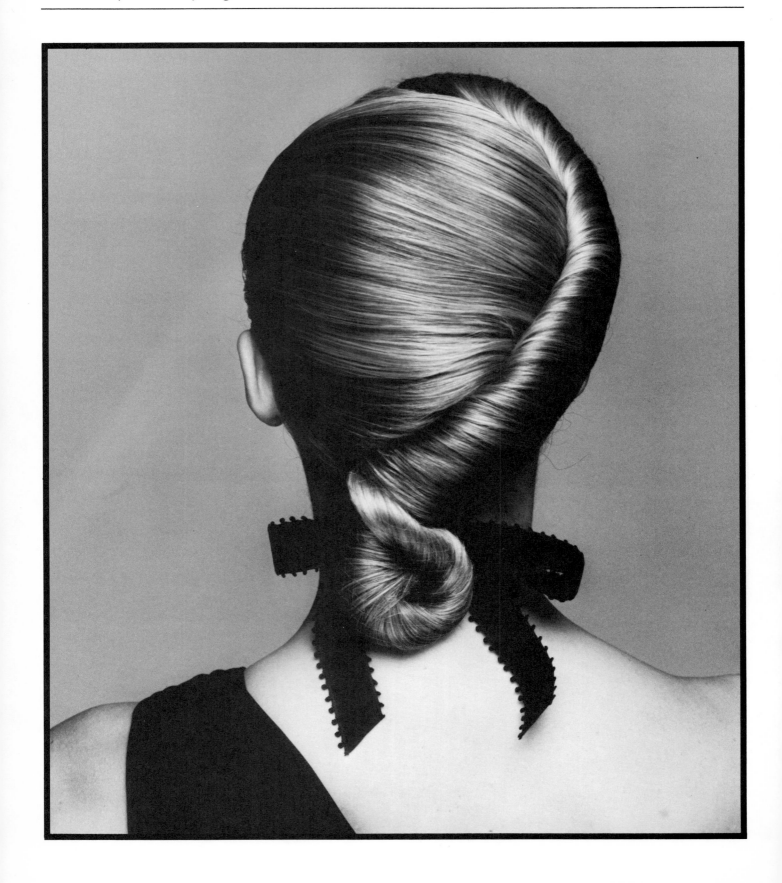

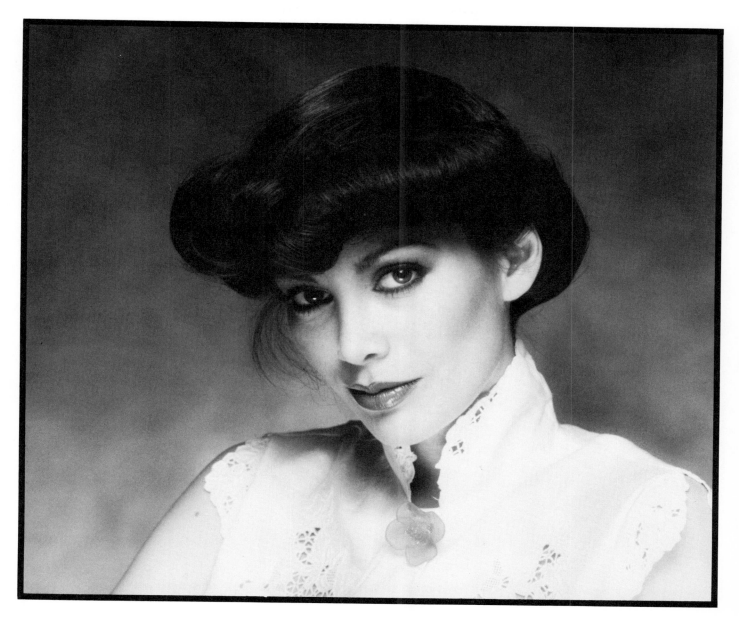

Opposite: For this asymmetrical twist, make a bobby-pinned base as you would for a French twist (see p. 70), and then start rolling from the forehead to the nape of the neck. Pin at the nape of the neck and twist the hair into a figure 8, tucking the ends under the roll.

Above: To make this kind of plump roll you will need to back-comb or use a filler of synthetic hair to create extra fullness. Start rolling from the nape of the neck to the forehead and right around to the nape again, then tuck the tail ends under the roll at the nape.

you don't have a rounded head shape, use a little back-combing at the crown before you start rolling to give a nice natural shape. If you do back-comb, smooth the back-combed hair with a bristle brush to create a rounded look, and then pin the back-combed area to the scalp about 1 or 2 inches from the bottom of your hairline. Smooth it out with a bristle brush.

Start rolling your hair in segments from the front. The size and volume of the roll and the segment is up to you. If you like plump rolls, you can back-comb the hair to be rolled here too, or use stuffing. (Stuffing, or filler, looks like hair and is made from plastic fibers and can be bought in dime stores or wig boutiques. Make sure the stuffing matches your hair color.) Use a bristle brush to smooth all the visible parts of the hair over the back-combing or stuffing, and then, starting at the forehead or in front of the ear, make sections as large as you want but no smaller than 2 inches, and begin to roll the hair as you would a thick piece of fabric. You will have a tail of hair left over. After you have made a roll, pin it in place with two or three hairpins, leaving the tail loose. You'll return later to anchor the roll more strongly. Then take the next section of hair, behind the ear, and incorporating the tail from the first section in with this section, begin to roll. Pin as above. Continue in this way until you reach the nape of the neck, leaving the last tail hanging out. Now begin to repeat rolling, starting at the other temple, until the rolls meet in the middle of the nape of your neck. You will have two tails left over from the rolls. Roll tails over your finger like a pin curl, and pin through roll so that pin is invisible.

Braiding

Somehow everybody seems to know how to make regular or pigtail braids. But there's a different kind of hair braiding, based on traditional corn-row and French braiding, which is a bit more

Right: The classic French braid is more difficult to do than simple pigtails, but it can be learned very quickly and is best and neatest when done on wet hair.

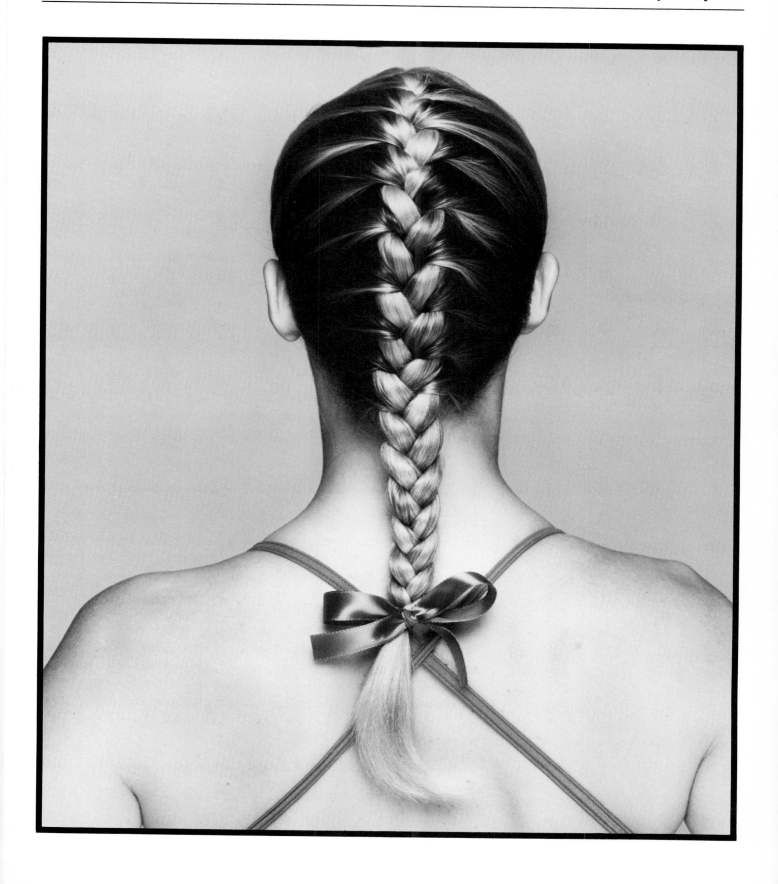

difficult to do. This kind of braiding differs from the better-known free-flying kind of pigtail braid in that it rests on the scalp. You may have seen marvelous, intricate corn-row braiding in magazines. The patterns can be simple or complex, and many times they approach an art form. To do these you really need another person to help you or you must be superhandy, so I'll just deal here with the basic techniques of French-braiding.

Take one section of hair and divide it into three parts. Begin to braid as you would a pigtail. After the first braid or twist, add hair that is not in that section from your scalp and work it into the braid. You will have a very thick braid that lies flat on your head. When you reach the bottom of your head, keep braiding as for a pigtail or stop there and make a ponytail with an elastic band or make a small chignon. No matter how thick your hair is when you reach the end of the braid, you will have flyaway hairs. It's best to make a chignon with the braid, tucking the tail under, or roll the braid back on itself and pin it to the scalp.

THE LONGEST TIME I SPENT ON A HAIR STYLE
In the Yucatán, I was inspired by a Mayan head. Marina Schiano, the model, agreed to let me work with her on it. I prepared for three hours the night before, making braids, hairpieces, ropes and twists, then I worked the whole next afternoon on Marina. I thought the very complicated hair style looked amusing, and the photographer did too. When we got to the top of a pyramid where we felt the shot would work well—it was 100 degrees and humid—we found a beehive. We had to be rather careful about this, especially since Marina was wearing only bracelets, rings, and her hair. That picture became a two-page spread in *Vogue* over ten years ago.

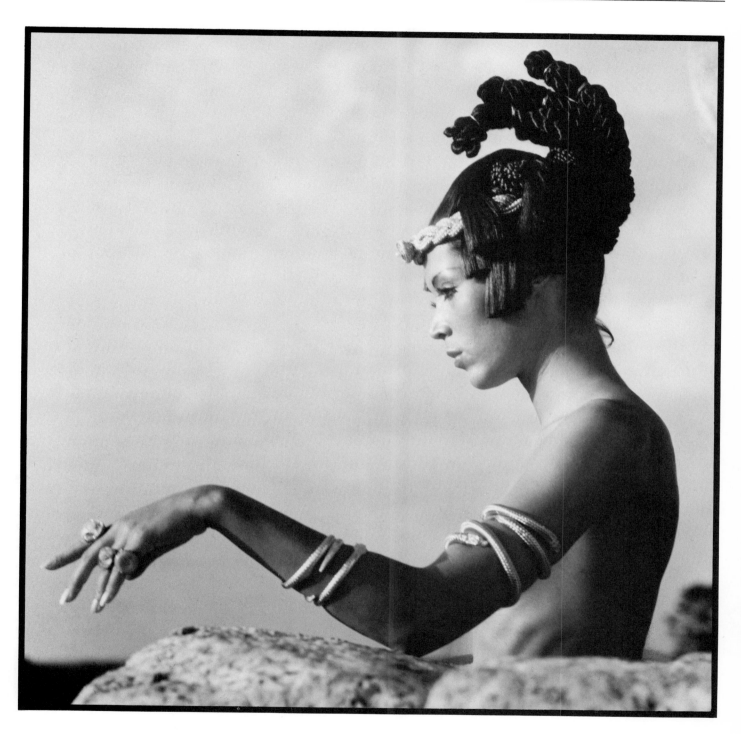

A Mayan-inspired head done on location
in Mexico. Photo: Suga

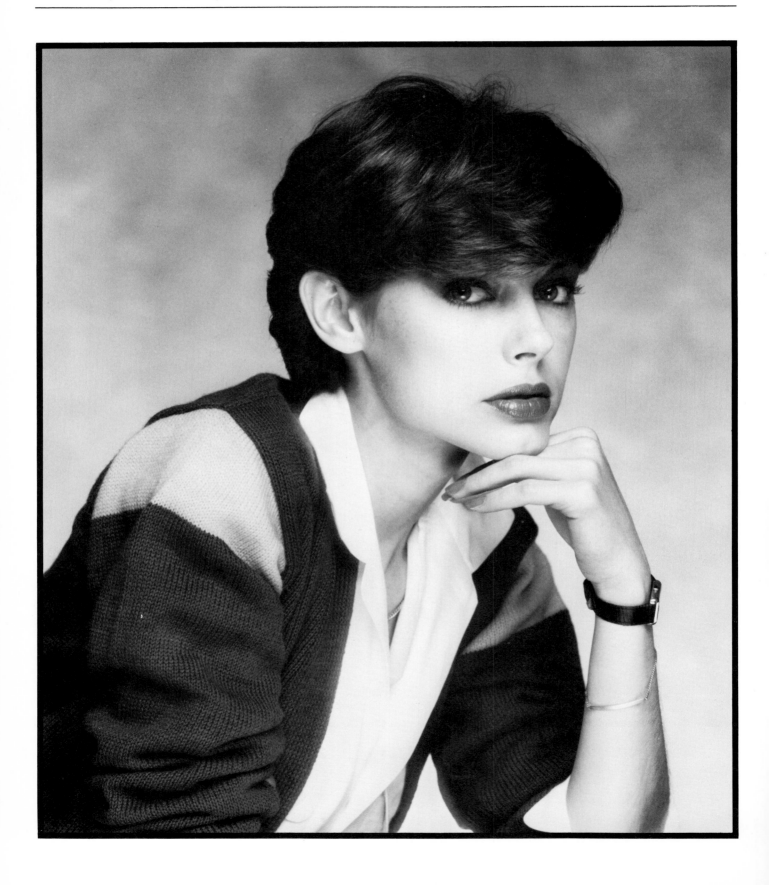

8

Your hair look:
theme and variations

A client of mine once told me that it took her years to find her own "look." She had followed fashion slavishly and had gone from short hair to long, from teased to straight to curly and back again, from colored to bleached to permanents to wigs and hairpieces. Finally she found a hairdresser in Paris who suggested that she try and live with her own hair texture and color and that she could even do her own hair and have it look attractive.

Left: Once you have established your basic look, you need some variations to keep it up-to-date and to keep yourself from getting bored with your hair.

Her hair is straight and fine and tends to go quite limp if there is any humidity in the air. She did not want to have to set her hair on rollers and she didn't want to be a slave to her hair in any way. Together she and her hairdresser worked out a classic center-part medium-length pageboy for her. She had a body wave to give her hair volume and to help maintain the line in all kinds of weather. She towel-dried her hair, and when it was almost dry she used a hand dryer and brush to give it fullness and to polish off the look. The total time expended on her hair, including a daily shampoo, was about twelve to fifteen minutes.

When she came to me she had had a pageboy look for almost two years and she explained to me that even though she felt she looked best with this style and that she could handle her own hair in a minimum amount of time, she was "just plain bored with it." Together we spent a great deal of time playing with her hair, putting it up in a knot, using combs, rolling it, changing the placement of the part, but to both of us nothing looked quite as attractive on her as the basic pageboy. Finally I decided to try out a very subtle variation of her turned-under pageboy.

I cut her hair about an inch all around the bottom, which would give her more bounce and then I layered the sides around her face to accentuate her cheekbones and to give her a bit more softness, as she had begun to wear softer clothes in keeping with the current fashion. Cutting an inch off and just layering the sides a bit are not very dramatic changes, but this was just enough for her to feel updated without being slavish to fashion and at the same time maintaining the basic shape and line of hair that were best suited to her and to her life style.

I often hear a woman who looks best with short hair say that there's not much she can do to change her look. She envies women with longer hair who can roll it or twist it into knots. In my experience many women, with short hair or long, feel they need a change of look every year and a half to two years. Short hair can easily adapt to a variety of looks, and my advice is: When you feel you want a new look, think in terms of slight or subtle changes that relate to or contrast with the kinds of clothes you are currently wearing. For example, if you like tailored skirts and blouses or simple pants with sweaters and blazers, then you might want to try a softer hair style to offset their severe effects.

Or perhaps you have had short, rather severe straight hair cut one length and parted on the side, and this is your "best look." You like to wear soft blouses and dresses, and your hair looks a bit *too* rigid for the softer lines of the clothing. To change your look and update it, you might consider eliminating the part (which is a straight, rather rigid line) and brushing your hair softly back, or you might think of having a body permanent to give a slight amount of wave and volume to your hair. Either change will be enough to make you feel you have something new, but neither will alter the basic look that you have established for yourself.

Perhaps you have short, layered hair which is naturally curly or has a permanent and which you have been finger-fluffing dry. You might try using a blow-dryer to straighten the line, or you can try brushing the forehead layer forward to make bangs if you don't already have them. If you have bangs, you might try brushing them off your face and fastening them with a small comb or barrette. Just by combing your hair forward off your forehead, you can make an interesting change in your look while maintaining the original line and length that look best on you.

Again, for short, layered hair (or for short, straight hair) you might try tucking your hair behind your ears if you have been wearing it in front or over the ears, and consider wearing larger or more important earrings. In the summer you can slick short hair back behind the ears and off the forehead with baby oil or hair conditioners, and you will have a very sleek, very chic look for the beach or patio. Remember that any time you comb your hair forward onto your face or brush it off your face you should take your jewelry and make-up into consideration.

Earrings, in particular, can add color and enhance the face when the hair is tucked behind the ears or pulled back.

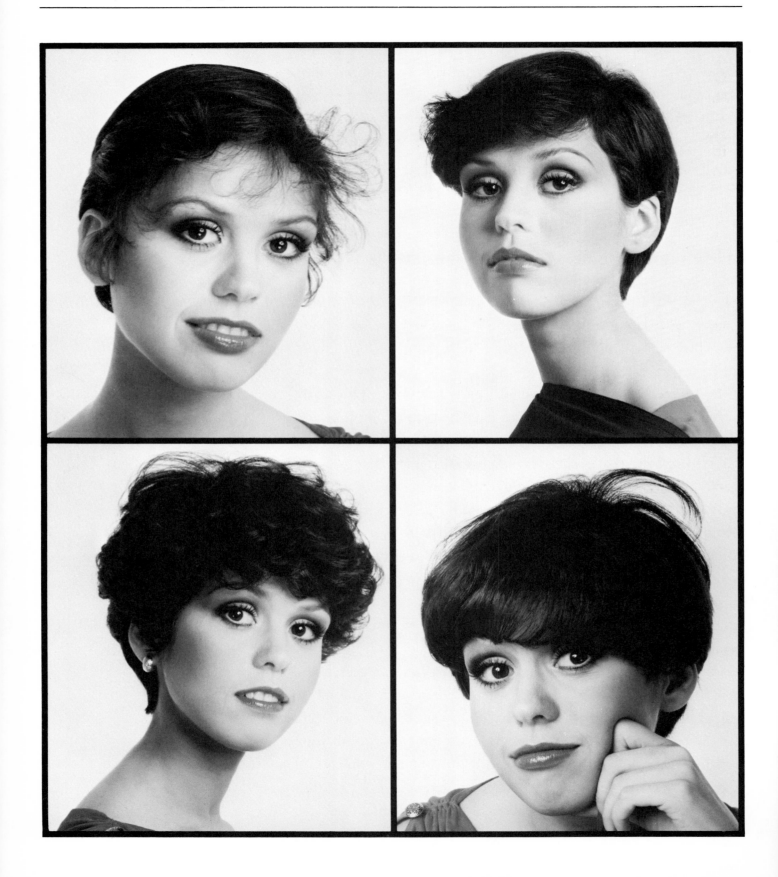

GOING ALL THE WAY

When Marie Osmond turned eighteen she decided she wanted a more adult image. On the night before she was to make an important commercial I went to her hotel to work with her on a new style. I'd sent her ten sketches for short hair, which is what I thought she needed to achieve a new look. She had shoulder-length hair when I arrived but she wasn't ready for short hair. So I cut it to chin length and she was very happy with it. The next day we started shooting. I felt the look of short hair was really necessary for what Marie was doing, so I pinned up the back to make it con-

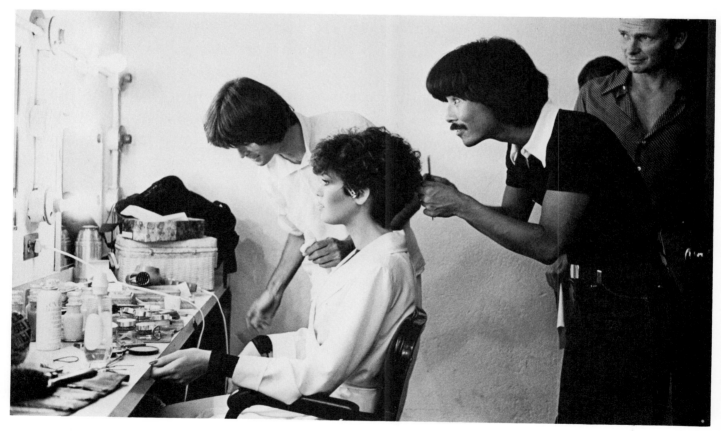

vincingly short for the cameras. The director (Richard Avedon) liked it, the dress designer (Bob Mackey) liked it, and finally Marie really liked it. So at lunchtime we decided to go all the way. That look was so successful that ever since I have flown regularly to Salt Lake City to trim her hair and her brother Donny's.

Opposite: 4 different looks for Marie. Photos: Avedon. *Above:* Behind the scenes, from left to right, make-up wizard Way Bandy, Marie, the author, Bob Mackey. Photo: Adrian Panaro.

If you have short hair, you might think of having your ears pierced if you have not already done so. Small studs—pearls, diamonds, turquoise—can add a spot of color and brilliance to the ears, and they add balance to short hair. Drop earrings and larger earrings should be worn with the shape of the head and the haircut in mind. I feel it's better to stay away from anything too long or too extreme for daytime, but generally, short hair lends itself better to all kinds and shapes of earrings.

Subtle alterations in make-up when made along with changes in hair style can add up to an interesting change in your look without being drastic. If you are wearing your hair off your face, think of emphasizing your eye make-up and intensifying your cheek color. The balance of the face is always changed by whether you wear your hair on or off your brow, or in front of or behind your ears. If your hair comes forward and you have thick bangs, be subtle about your make-up and use a light hand—there is a lot going on around your face, and you don't want to overdo. If your hair is off your face or slicked back for the summer, try experimenting with more defined eyes by contouring or intensifying the eye shadow that you normally use. If you have had your hair cut from long to short and your hair is dark, you may find that it looks even darker because it is framing your face in a new way. A change in make-up will help balance your new look. Think of toning down your make-up if your hair is on your forehead, or giving it extra emphasis if it is short and combed back.

Whether the change in your hair style is big or small, it's important always to think about changes in make-up. I suggest that you take the time to have a private lesson with a make-up artist or visit one or two of the cosmetics counters in your local department store to have a make-up consultation.

To try and give you some idea of what you can do to change your look without losing the basic line and length that you have established for yourself, I've made the following list of basic haircuts with some simple modifications. Many of the modifications you can quickly and easily do yourself.

Long straight hair

Simple, stick-straight long hair is usually a good look for a girl or a very young woman. However, there are many ideas that you can use to make this look more sophisticated and interesting. A body perm will give more volume and bounce to your hair, and makes it easier to turn the ends up or under into a pageboy. The sides can be layered to give softness. If you decide on shaping or layering the sides, you can use pin curls or rollers to give direction and curl to this area. Cutting bangs if you don't already have them will give you quite a different look. Try giving bangs direction and fullness by rolling them on sponge rollers when you are drying your hair after a shampoo.

Twisting a strand of hair from the temple to behind the ear adds softness and interest. You can anchor the twist with a barrette or clip or small flower. Twist strands at each temple for a variation on this theme, then have both twists meet in the back and pin together with a small ornament.

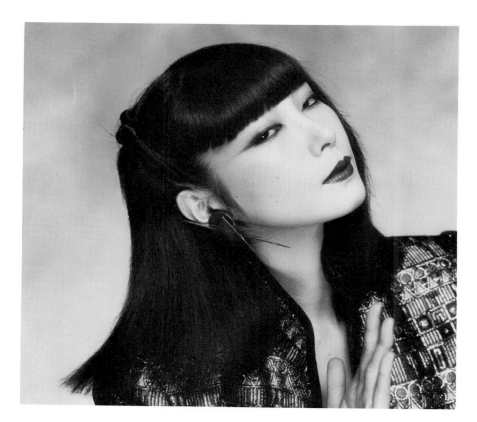

It's easy to become bored with long straight hair. You can make major changes in your basic look, e.g., by cutting bangs, or minor ones like twisting strands or making little knots.

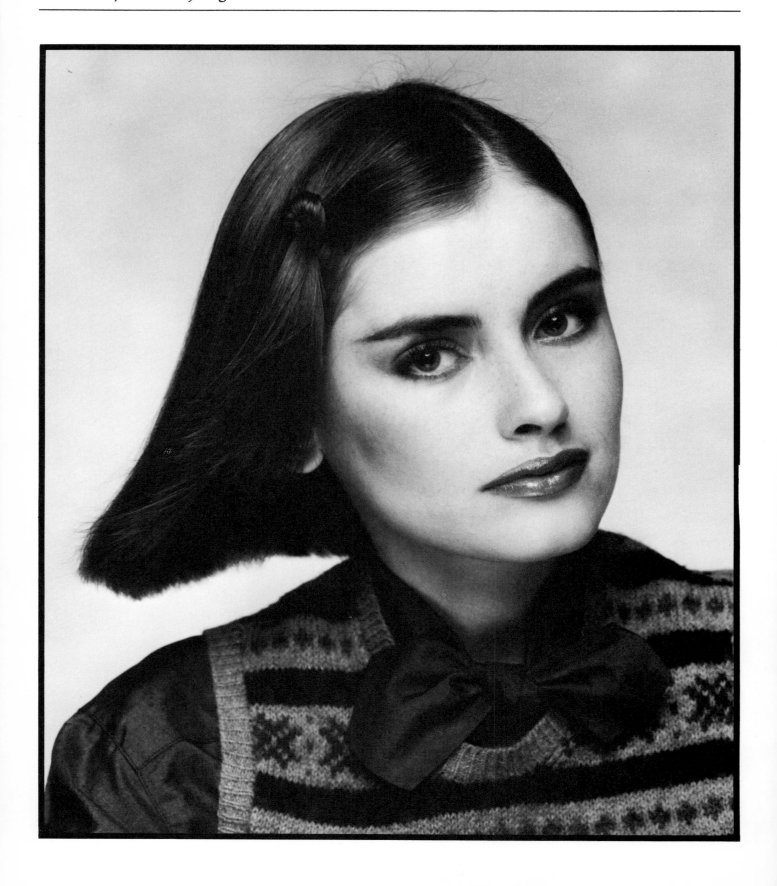

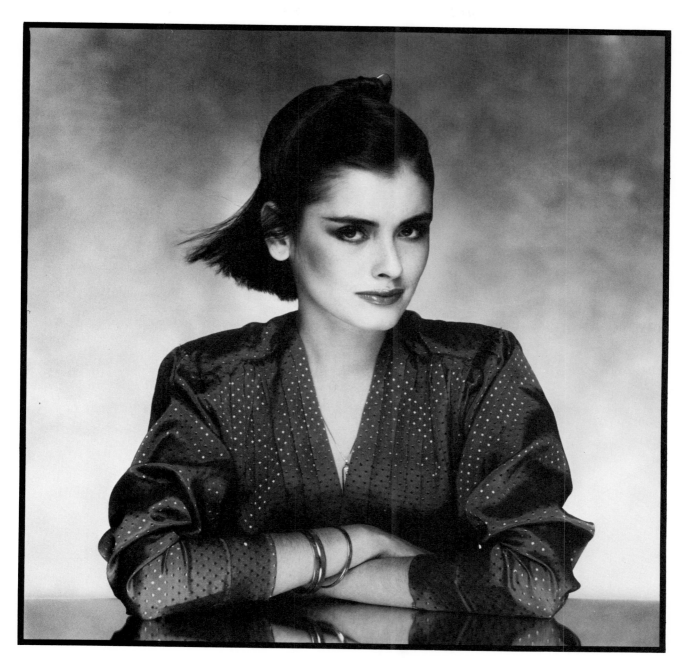

Above: A nighttime variation for medium-length very fine hair. (The looks on both pages are based on the same one-length haircut.) Take hair from sides and front and twist to center of crown. Twist hair again into a chignon or knot and anchor with a comb or decorative barrette.

Left: A daytime variation for medium-length very fine hair. To keep hair off the face you can always make a little braid or use a pretty comb or barrette with this kind of cut. But here is a new kind of knot: Take hair and knot like a piece of rope, slipping the end of hair through itself, making a loop and pulling it tight. Anchor securely with a bobby pin underneath.

Long wavy or curly hair

If you want to straighten your hair at times, use the wrapping technique described on page 56. If your hair is all one length, try having it cut into longish layers to give it more shape and movement. Experiment with twisting strands as for Long Straight Hair, above. Another pretty and classic look for your hair is achieved by taking hair from the forehead to the crown, and then pulling it smoothly back off the forehead into a pony-tail. Secure the ends with a coated elastic band and fasten to the back of the head with a pretty comb. The contrast of the smooth crown and the full wavy hair is attractive, and this look goes well with almost any clothes you wear.

Combs work well with long wavy or curly hair because they anchor into it easily. If you have coarse, thick hair you can use larger combs with thicker teeth. If you have fine hair, stick to combs that have narrowly spaced thin teeth. Try combing your hair back from the temples and setting combs above the ears. Or if you have a side part, just use one comb placed in the same way for an interesting asymmetrical effect. If you have a problem with combs falling out, run a bobby pin at right angles over the lower portion of the teeth; this should lock the comb in place.

Medium-length straight hair

This is the best length for a classic pageboy. If you are tired of the turned-under look, try blow-drying the ends up. A body wave will give you volume and help maintain the shape and line. A partial permanent on only the ends will help give you a sleek stay-in-place turned-under or flipped-up look.

The way you treat the sides of your hair will give you interesting variations on the basic look. Try layering the sides and rolling them off your face. Or try the reverse and blow-dry the layers toward the face to frame and accentuate your cheekbones. Think of having a partial permanent on the side pieces; this can help to maintain line and direction of the hair so that you don't have to use rollers or curling irons.

Take strands of hair from the side layers, starting at the temples, then wrap them with fine silk cord or thin pieces of leather and secure each behind your ears with a hairpin. Make one tie only if you have a side part, or make two if you part in the center; have them meet and twist them together at the back of your head.

You might try making one or more small braids from side strands. When you unbraid them you'll find you have finely waved hair, which looks interesting as a contrast to your normally straight hair.

You can change the balance of this length of hair by making it shorter in the back and longer in the front. Or you can have the sides shorter and the back longer or the hair can be cut evenly all around. You can layer straight medium-length hair, but I advise against it unless you intend to have a body wave or regular permanent. Straight layers tend to hang there without much bounce, and unless you have some wave, your hair can end up looking choppy and lifeless.

Medium-length wavy or curly hair

You have a choice of layering your hair or keeping it all one length. I often suggest layering because with the weight of the hair cut off, it can curl up more easily. If your hair is wavy and you want more curl, you might consider a permanent. A perm will work best on layered hair because it's easier to make curls if the hair is not too long. You might try a partial permanent at the crown to give you more height should you need it. If you have fine, limp hair, consider having a body perm to give you manageability and to intensify the wave that's already there.

You can also easily use combs and barrettes in your hair. If your hair is wavy and full, try to show the shape of your head to give the proper balance and proportion to the rest of your body.

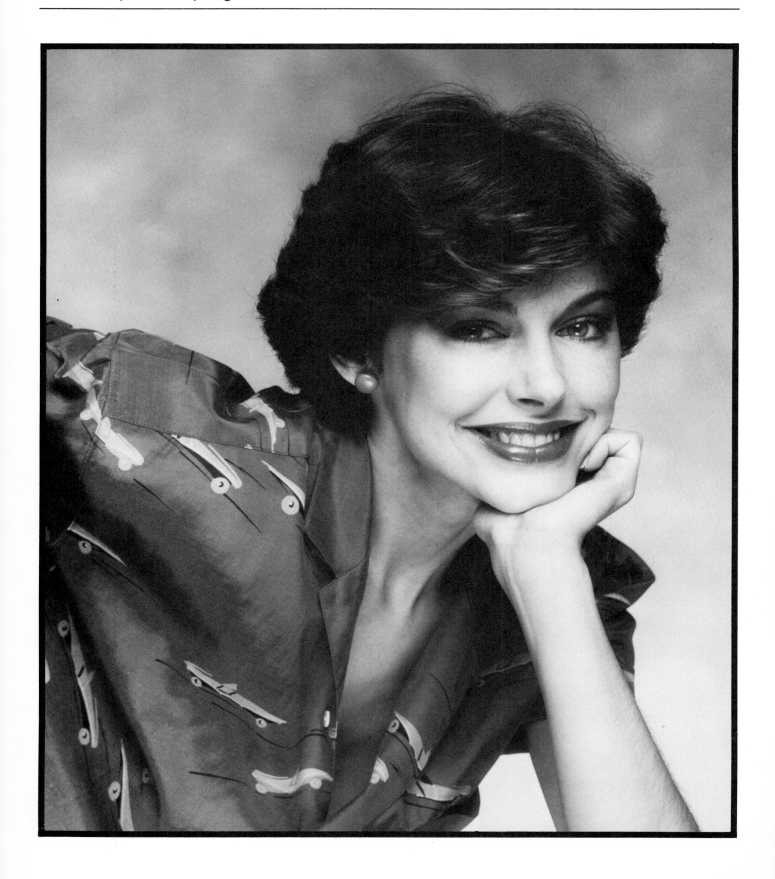

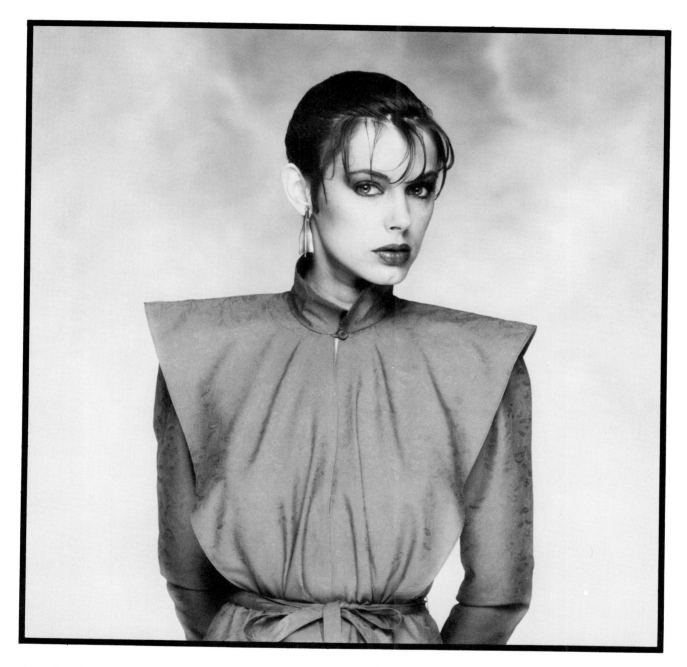

Opposite: This is a basic layered haircut for short, slightly wavy hair. All it needs for maintenance is washing and fluff-drying with your fingers. If you feel you don't have enough volume, you could try having a very gentle body perm. For the quickest variation on this look, simply tuck hair behind your ears (p. 88).

Above: For a dramatic evening look based on the same haircut as on the opposite page, you must start with wet hair and work a gel-type setting lotion into it. (I use Dep lotion or Dippity-Do.) Comb hair straight back, pull out some wisps and do not touch again! Remember, earrings and make-up become more important when hair is so severe.

Try combing your hair sleekly off the temples, and firmly anchor combs about 3 or 4 inches off the face. The flat, combed-back portion of your hair makes a nice contrast with the loose, curly areas. Rolling and twisting the sides and front of your hair will also show the shape of your head.

Short straight hair

Short straight hair can be cut all one length or it can be shaped at the neck and sides to softly frame the face and head. There are many basic variations for short straight hair. You can wear it brushed off or brushed toward the face, or in front of or behind the ears. You can have bangs cut straight across or cut in a more casual zigzag manner, or you can have bangs that taper down the temple toward the ears. To make a change, simply brush bangs back and secure with a pretty comb or two if you need to.

Making a part or changing its placement can also yield a new look. Sometimes just by changing the placement of a part you will notice more fullness or volume because you are brushing in the direction opposite to the natural growth pattern, and the hairs are lifted up and out from the roots.

Each of the changes I've talked about results in a very different look. Try experimenting with all of them, keeping in mind what I said before about jewelry and make-up.

If you need volume, consider a body wave to give you softness and fullness without curl.

Short straight hair can look very different in the summer or when you are on vacation. Put baby oil or a hair conditioner on your hair, then comb it and slick it back into a sleek, shiny cap. This is a good look for the pool or beach and is one of the best ways of protecting hair from sunburn.

Short curly or wavy hair

Short curly or wavy hair is usually cut in layers, and you can see quite a difference in your look just by changing the direction of the way the hair usually lies. Brushing layers forward over the forehead makes full thick bangs; brushing in the other direction, off the face, can give a more sophisticated feeling. Brushing the hair in front of or over your ears accentuates the cheekbones, and brushing it back behind the ears opens up the face and generally gives more emphasis to the eyes and mouth. If you brush or comb your hair in the direction that it grows, try reversing the direction—it will give you an extra lift.

Short curly or wavy hair is a good candidate for partial permanents. You can set rollers or rods on the crown for added height and volume or use them at the hairline to make the ends of hair turn down or under. You can use a partial permanent to change the direction of a wave or to recurl an unruly or unmanageable portion of hair.

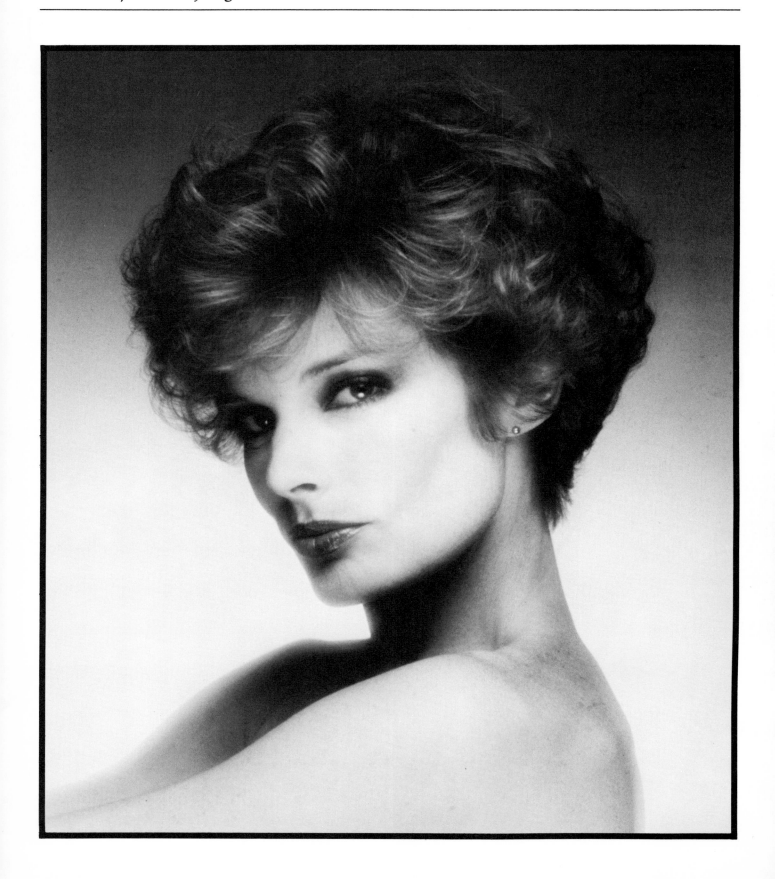

9

A word about age

I basically feel that no matter what your age, any hair style is appropriate if it looks right on you and you are comfortable with it. However, there are times when I see a woman who is trying to look younger perhaps by wearing her hair straight or wavy about 3 or more inches below her shoulders. This is obviously a style more appropriate for someone under thirty or thirty-five than it is to a more mature woman. If a woman is *obviously* trying to look younger, it's not working—it's too obvious.

As a woman gets older she must reassess and re-evaluate her hair in terms of color and style because the structure of the face

Left: If you have gray hair, keep it very full and soft. Teasing and spraying look rigid; try a perm instead. Wear hair swept up so that your face has a lift.

is subtly changing. If you are wearing long straight hair, take a good look at yourself in the mirror. If your hair hangs down straight, is it bringing your face down too? This is the most common problem with long hair on someone who's over fifty. When the face and jawline tend to become less firm, straight long hair can accentuate the problem. You can still wear hair to the shoulder, but I strongly advise clearing the area around the jawline and ear by cutting or curling the hair in these areas shorter or by rolling or twisting it off the face.

A word of caution if you have long gray hair and wear it in a bun or rolled up. If you wear your hair this way, your clothes and accessories must be fashionable or you run a risk of looking old-fashioned or matronly. Gray hair in a bun or twist can look extremely attractive with a soft silk shirt and tweed skirt or a glamorous dress, but it can have an aging effect with an out-of-date pantsuit or carelessly put together separates.

After a certain age, fifty or thereabouts, I prefer the look of short, perfectly cut hair for a woman. To me this looks very chic and smart. Hair should have a certain amount of volume, and again, the line from the temple to chin should be clear and hair swept softly off the face. Gray hair, in particular, looks good when it's short and gently curled, and I stress that it must be well cut to take advantage of any natural curl or wave.

If your hair is short and straight, it may be too extreme. If your face is too full or too thin, you will need some kind of volume to your hair to balance and soften your face. I would suggest a body wave or a permanent to correct this, but if your hair is colored or bleached be careful: gray hair that has been overly frosted can be troublesome with a permanent because it is more difficult to predict results and degree of curl. Make sure you consult with both your colorist and your hairdresser before you have a permanent.

If you are completely gray and you want to color your hair, think of the gray as a base color and add darker or lighter tones to it. Don't tint or bleach more than one or two shades, as your hair may turn out looking unnatural and obviously colored. If you really prefer dark hair, keep some gray around the face at the hairline and at the part. Think of the gray as frosting or highlighting the darker portions of your hair.

SERVICE ENTRY

Quite often in rich ladies' apartment buildings I have a hard time getting in and I am asked to enter through the service door. Many times I am asked if I am a TV repairman or an air-conditioner fixer, as I carry my equipment in a bag and I don't get too dressed up.

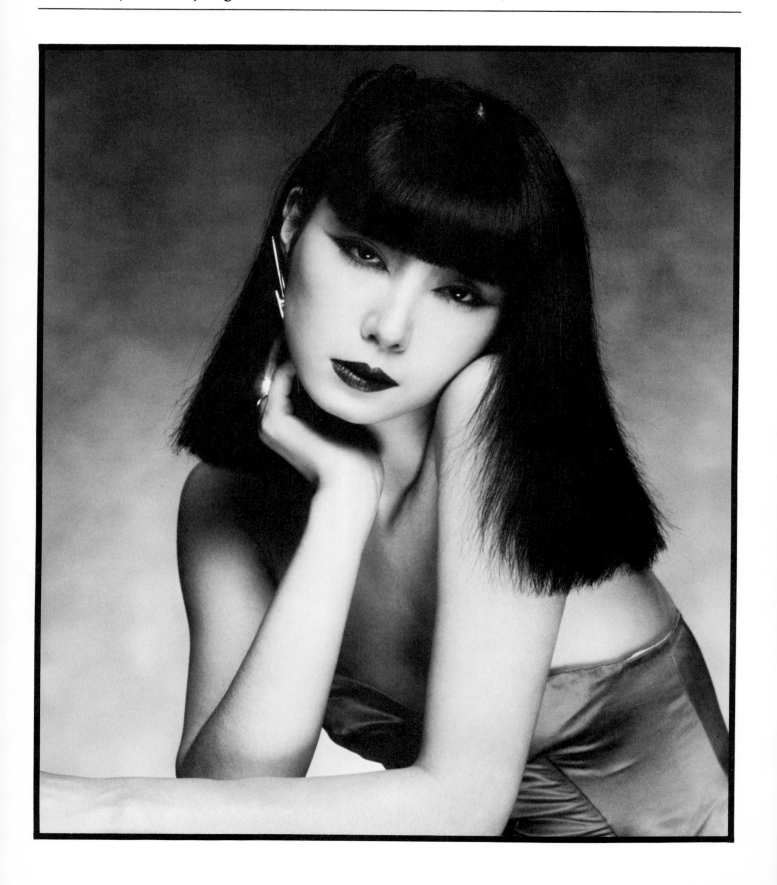

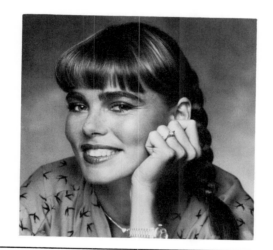

10

How to cut your own bangs

I really don't believe in home haircutting for one major reason— and it's not because I feel hair can only be done by professionals. I *do* think hair should be handled and cut by those who know best, but the reason I'm not advocating home cutting is that you can't see the back of your head, so you'll never be able to achieve the perfect shape and balance that, ideally, the professional can do for you.

However, you *can* see your bangs, so it becomes easy to cut them yourself. Many people think bangs grow faster than other

Bangs should be cut at least every week to ten days and it's very easy to learn how. Sayoko *(left)* and Margaux Hemingway *(above)* show perfect examples of beautiful bangs.

hairs on the head, but it's really not true. It appears that your bangs grow faster because they are close to or almost covering your eyes, and it seems that you can see them grow millimeter by millimeter. To keep your bangs in perfect shape they need trimming every seven to ten days.

Pin all your hair back except your bangs. Leaving bangs dry, comb them forward and shake your head so they are softly in place and not plastered to your forehead. Now estimate how much you want to take off. The amount should not exceed more than ¼ or ⅓ inch; ½ inch is too much.

Wet bangs. Make a section from temple to temple, going about ½ inch in from your forehead. Pin back the rest of your bangs, and divide this forehead section into vertical thirds. Starting with the center section, hold the hair between your index and third fingers and bring it straight down to the top of your nose. Then cut ¼ inch only, straight across. Do not cut where you think the bangs should go, cut ¼ inch or, at most, ⅓ inch.

Take one of the side sections and a bit of the cut-off front section. If you want straight-across bangs, cut the side section straight across, using the hair from the center section as a guide to the length. If you like the sides of your bangs longer (or shorter), cut the side section on the angle that you prefer. Repeat this same process for the other side section.

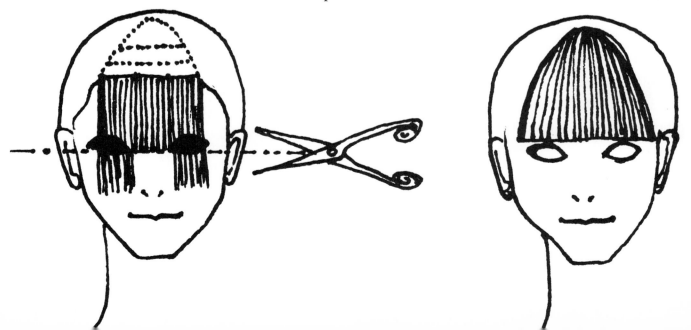

Now go to the hair that you have pinned back. Make another ½-inch section or layer parallel to the first one that you have just cut. Repeat the same process, remembering that this layer should be just a little bit longer than the first layer—and I mean just a little! These first two layers give you a guide; if you have other layers to your bangs, just follow the same procedure, making each layer no more than a millimeter or two longer than the one that preceded it. If you like zigzag or shaggy bangs, you should use the same layering procedure, and cut mini-sections at slight angles.

MUSICAL BANGS

Seiji Ozawa, the conductor, and his wife are good friends of mine. Both like to wear their hair rather long. Since they are traveling around the world a great deal of the time, it is often difficult for us to get together.

Since the front of Seiji's hair cannot be too long because he must be able to see when he's conducting, I've taught his wife how to cut his bangs, and he can go for about three months without a haircut. He'll stand still to let me cut his hair, but he never stops moving for his wife, who has a difficult time with him. She, however, is quite fussy and refuses to let him reciprocate with the bang-cutting.

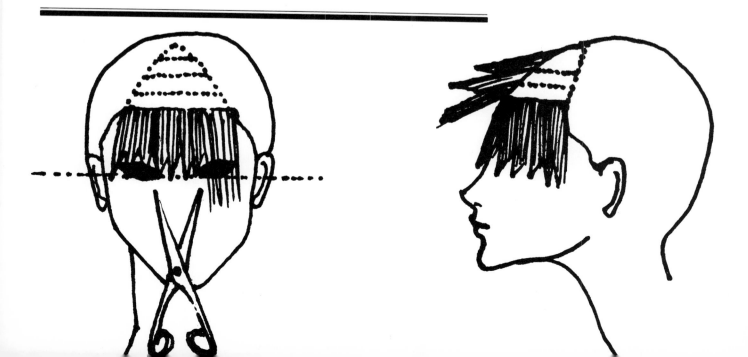

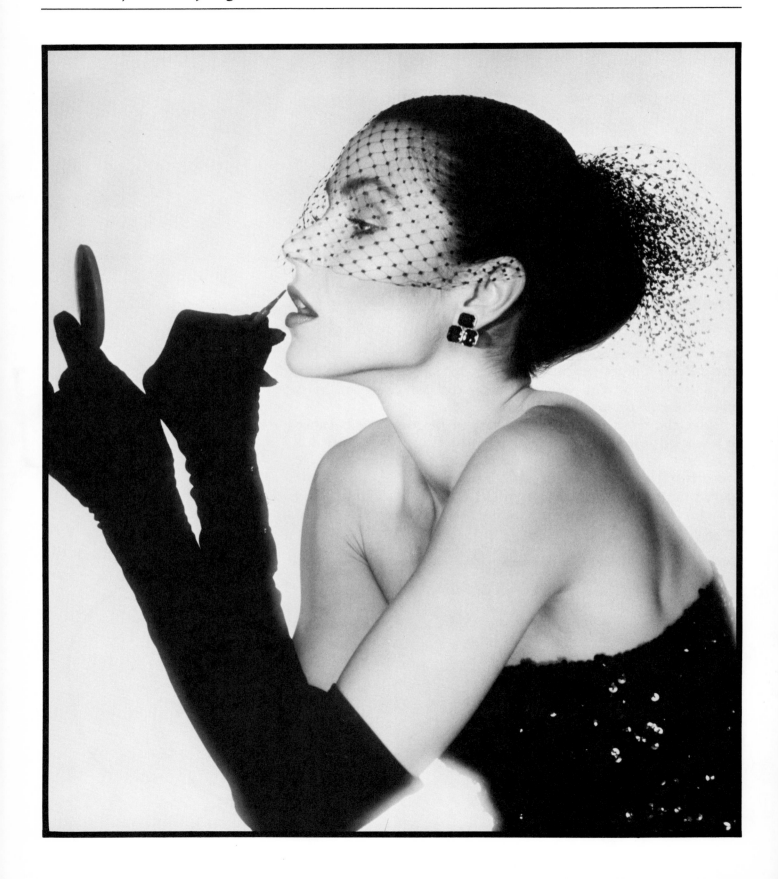

11

Instant glamour:
tricks of the trade
and special effects

Most of us who do a great deal of work with fashion magazines and television have developed a bag of tricks that we use to give instant glamour. Often, on location, a rain cloud can be seen coming and the photographer will say, "Quick, the light is going, do something!" What he usually means is that he wants a change in the look that's already on the model and he's hoping that the change might just "make the picture." Also, for some

Left: When you use a veil the look of the head must be small. See p. 124.

photographic shootings, the hair must be superperfect, no hair-pins can show, each hair must be in place, the chignon must make a perfect figure eight with not a millimeter of extra bulge on either side, or the flower must be placed just so, or the braid must lie absolutely flat. There are ways and means of adapting these effects for home use, and also tricks to giving yourself instant glamour for a special evening out when you have no more than ten minutes to fiddle with your hair and you want to look special.

Quick tricks

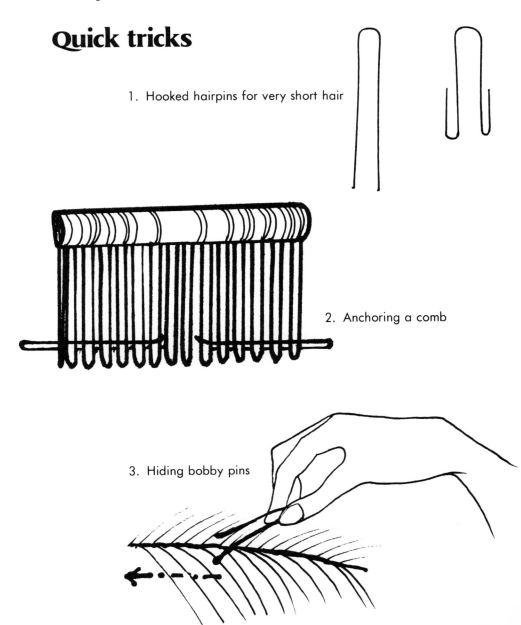

1. Hooked hairpins for very short hair

2. Anchoring a comb

3. Hiding bobby pins

Smoothing stick-out hair

Slightly dampen a cotton ball with hair spray or lotion, or rub it gently in pomade and smooth it over the fine hairs, and they will stay neatly in place.

To beat the static electricity

Spray a bristle brush with hair spray and lightly brush the top layers of your hair. If your hair is very flyaway from static electricity, spray the brush and run it gently through your hair. Hairs will lie smoothly in place.

Holding hairpins in short hair

If your hair is too short to hold a hairpin and you want to keep down an unruly tuft, take the smallest and finest hairpin and bend one or both of its tips to make a small hook. If you stick this into your hair, it won't come out because it is hooked into the hair and cannot slip. (1)

Anchoring a comb

Place the comb in your hair at the angle you want it. Then run a bobby pin at right angles to the comb under the top layer of your hair, just catching the ends of the teeth of the comb. (2)

Hiding a bobby pin

Always place the pin parallel to the edge of the roll or twist or braid and insert it into the roll. (3)

Special effects

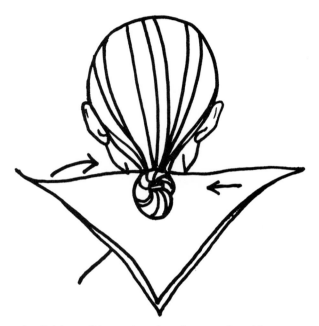

1. Fold scarf into triangle, place under chignon.

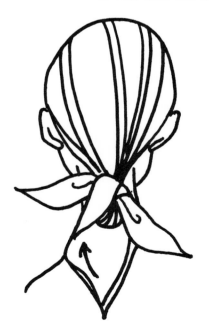

2. Tie left and right ends together, then cover chignon with last end.

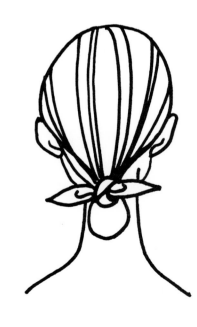

3. Tie end pieces together again and tuck any extra fabric into knot.

Invisible hair net

The invisible hair net works to keep chignons or knots perfectly smooth, and to make the short hairs stay in place. When you make a knot, use four or five big hairpins to hold it momentarily in place. Then take the finest hair net that matches your hair color and cover the knot with it, tucking the unused part of the net under the knot or chignon. Now take the pins out one by one, re-anchoring each pin over the net at the base of the knot, thereby securing it firmly with very few pins.

Achieving volume with fillers

Whenever you don't have enough volume or fullness for your hair, use fillers or stuffing (available at most wig shops). Fillers look like real hair and are made from synthetic fibers. Be sure to match the color of the filler to the color of your hair. Cut or pull off a bit of the filler, and if you are rolling the hair, roll hair around the filler, anchoring it with hairpins. If you are making a chignon, secure the filler with pins where you will be placing the chignon, and place the chignon over the filler.

You can also pin filler at the crown of your head and roll hair over it to give a beautifully rounded shape to the head.

The envelope trick

Make a ponytail and fasten it with a coated elastic band. Fold a small scarf or handkerchief into a triangle. Keeping the point of the triangle facing downward, place the scarf underneath the ponytail (1) and tie (2) a small envelope covering the whole ponytail. (3) Secure with bobby pins. If you use a small silk handkerchief, the look can be very dressy and is most attractive on a summer evening. See illustrations left.

How to make a very soft knot or Gibson Girl

First, make a giant pin curl, about 2 inches in diameter, where you want your knot to go. Secure this with two crisscrossed bobby pins. Brush all your hair into one hand at the top of your head, holding this hank of hair about 2 to 5 inches away from your scalp. (1) Place a coated elastic band where you are gripping the hair. Then push the elastic band to where the pin curl is. (2) This should give a wonderful soft droop to the hair. Now secure the elastic band to the pin curl with one or two hairpins. Roll or twist the tail over your fingers into a small knot and secure this in place. (3)

Right: Jane Lee Salmons looks superglamorous in an asymmetrical Gibson. *Below:* 1. Put your head down and hold hair about 2 to 5 inches from scalp. 2. Push hair into pin-curl base, pin down. 3. Twist tail over base and pin in place.

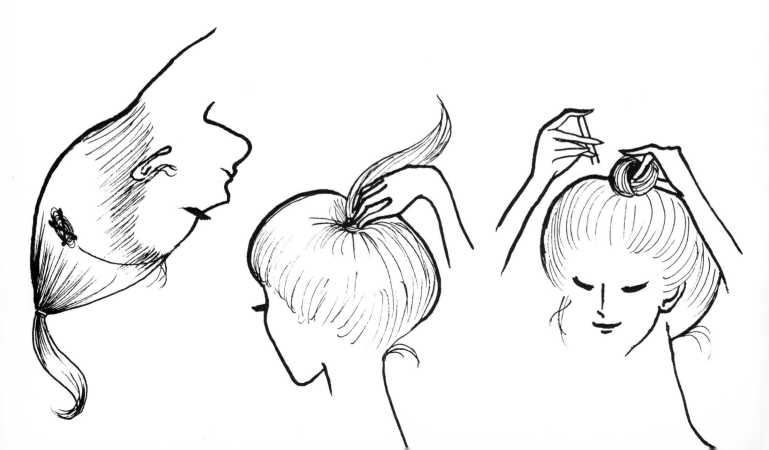

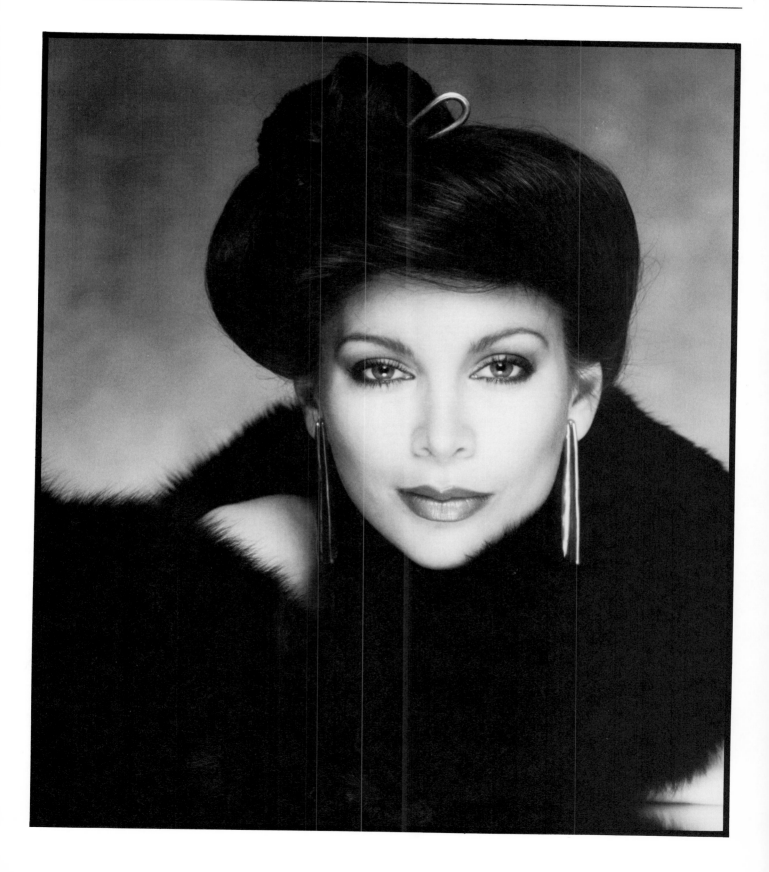

Combs, clips and barrettes

The main reason to use a comb, a clip or a barrette is to *hold* the hair. Don't put any of these where they don't make sense—that is, don't place them arbitrarily. Even if you are using a comb for decoration, it should make sense by holding the hair. Secure the comb in the opposite direction from which you want the hair to go. The most popular combs and barrettes are black and tortoise shell, but there are many colors you can enjoy. I particularly like red and gold, and I usually stay away from pastel colors. I recommend the lightest-weight comb possible because it stays better in the hair. If your comb doesn't stay in place, run a bobby pin at right angles to it, just catching the edges of the teeth. Then comb the top layer of hair over it.

Flowers

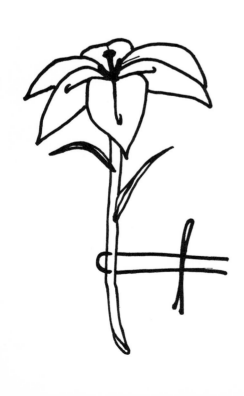

I like to use fresh flowers in the hair—white gardenias, smallish orchids or lilies, freesia and anemones, and tropical flowers such as hibiscus and bougainvillaea. Be sure to take the pistil out of the flower, as the pollen can stain your clothing.

When you put flowers in your hair, please think of balance and the proportions of what you're wearing. Don't forget to include jewelry in your assessment—sometimes a flower and jewelry are just too much together.

Sporty clothes and tailored wear do not usually lend themselves to flowers. Romantic dresses, evening clothes and softer looks are more appropriate.

If the flower is very big, please put it away from the face or to the back of the head. Sometimes a flower tends to dominate the face. Keep the stem short, but long enough to pin. If it is a small flower, a bobby pin will usually do the trick. If it is larger—an orchid or lily perhaps—pierce the stem with a hairpin and use a bobby pin perpendicular to the hairpin to secure it.

Right: Unexpected touch—grape leaves in Rene Russo's hair. Photo, courtesy of Revlon. Photographer: Avedon.

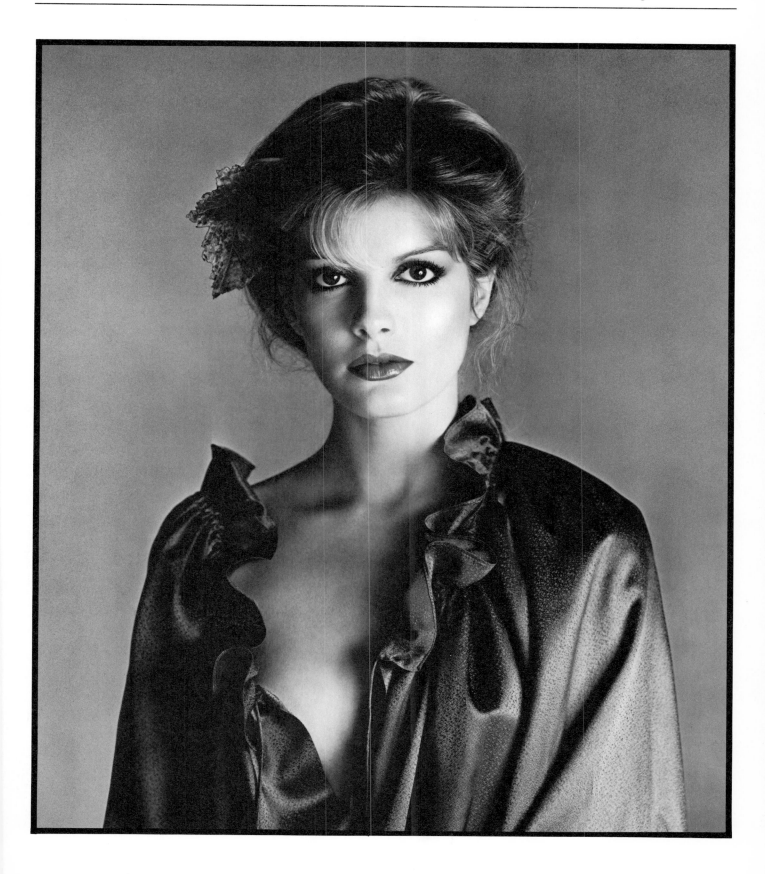

Of course you can use artificial flowers if you like them. I think silk is prettiest and most flattering to the face. I'd suggest staying away from plastic flowers, as they are too artificial-looking—use combs or clips or ribbons instead.

Ribbons

Ribbons and bows are symbolic of romance, and there are many ways of using them. There are two basic techniques in dealing with bows: the first is to make a separate bow and attach it to the ribbon with bobby pins, and the second is to make a bow with the ribbon itself. If you are not terrific with bows, I suggest that you employ the first method.

The variations of ribbon use are limited only by your imagination. Fashion magazines often have interesting styles using ribbons. Try braiding ribbons into your hair—you can use the ribbon as a separate strand or mix it with one of the braiding strands. You can twist ribbons into your hair and you can use them as ties (these techniques are discussed on page 75). The image of a woman with ribbons in her hair does not necessarily have to be girlish. Black satin ribbons give an elegant effect, and when they are wrapped into a chignon they are extremely sophisticated.

Jewels

Aesthetically I do not like to put expensive or large jewelry on the head, although I have done so. Once I put a diamond-and-pearl necklace into the back of a chignon, but this was a rare occasion. Usually a woman wears earrings and often a necklace, and if, in addition, she puts something in her hair, the effect can be overdone. If you do put a jewel in your hair, you must anchor it securely (and please take out insurance!). The best way to anchor it is with crisscrossed bobby pins.

Right: You can have a sophisticated grown-up look with ribbons. "Clinique Photo" of Maura McGagney by Barry Lategan.

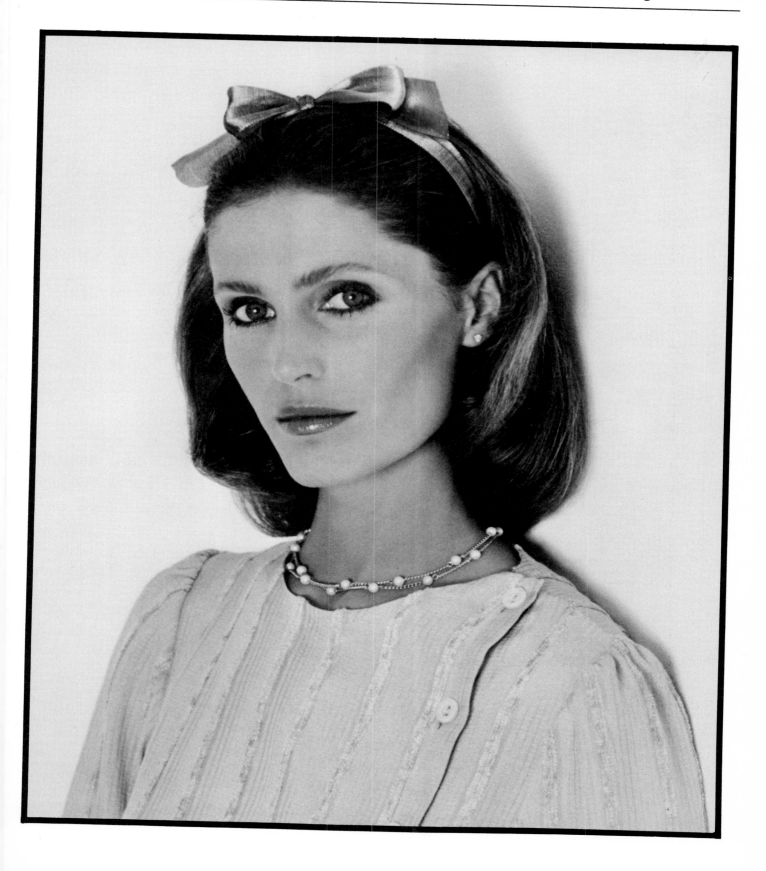

Sticks

Sticks must be placed in chignons or knots; otherwise they make no sense. I prefer to use them in chignons or knots at the crown or at the back of the head and I use a variety of materials—gold, silver, ivory, woods, bamboo and plastic are attractive. They give a special look, and I suggest them primarily for evening use when you might want something dramatic and sophisticated.

Feathers

I suggest these only for evening, and usually for dramatic effect. Never use large feathers because you'll look like a show girl or a bird. Usually feathers are attached to small combs which are easy to manage. If they don't come with a comb or pin and the stem of the feather is too thick, pierce the stem with a hairpin and anchor the hairpin with the bobby pin.

Veils

A simple veil can be used to great effect. I like the look of a veil over the eyes with a small bow in the back. When you use a veil, the hair should be slick and the look of the head should be small. Aesthetically I prefer that a veil go no lower than the tip of your nose unless you are on a strict diet or trying not to smoke, in which cases it is allowable to let the veil be longer.

Right: Singer and model Beverly Johnson has an all-out glamorous look for evening. All her hair has been twisted tightly to the top of her head and pinned with shiny feathers.

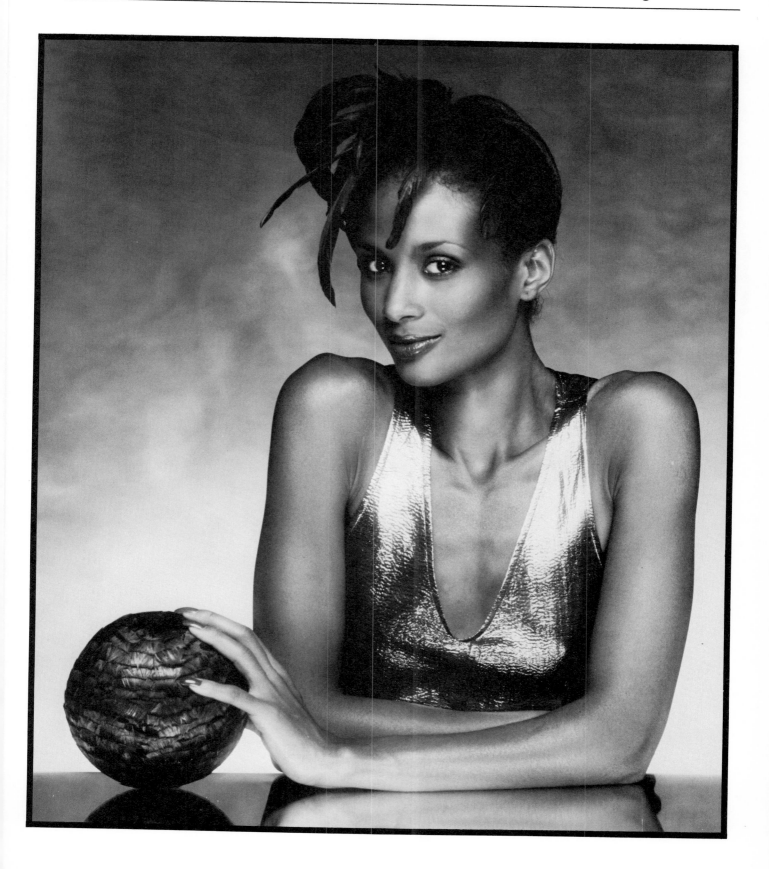

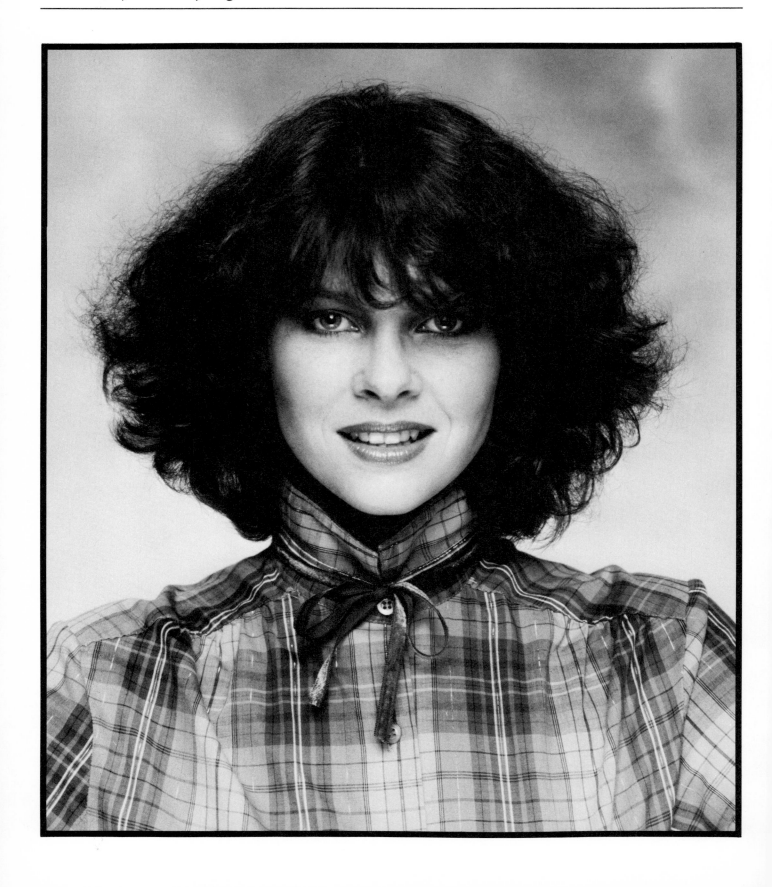

12

All about permanents

"Permanent" is a very tricky word. People use it in many different ways and with a variety of meanings. Basically, a permanent changes the degree of curl and the texture of your hair. For example, straight hair can become wavy or curly, or fine hair can be given more body.

When you have a permanent, your hair is rolled on rods or rollers in various widths. Different chemical solutions are applied to set the hair into a "permanent" wave or curl which will last from three to seven months, depending on the strength of the permanent and the rate of growth of the hair. Hair can also be

There's a whole new world in permanents. You can perm all of your hair or just parts of it. *Left:* A partial permanent that waves only the ends, not the roots.

"permanently" straightened by chemical solutions, but of course, as the hair grows, it will come out naturally curly.

Many people feel that permanents make kinks or frizz or damage the hair. This is not necessarily true. The technology of permanents has changed radically in the past few years; the chemicals or solutions have been reformulated and are loaded with conditioners to keep the hair supple and healthy. Today permanents, if they are carefully administered with the proper solutions, can even be given on bleached or colored hair with no bad effects.

We are also using permanents in many new ways. We can perm different parts of the hair to give differet looks and to solve many hair problems. Permanents can give volume and fullness to fine, limp hair, and they can give body to hair that needs line and shape. They can help to tame coarse, unruly hair, and as I said, they can even straighten hair. Certainly today's perm is nothing like the old crimped ones our grandmothers used to get.

At least a third of my clients have permanents, although you'd never know it, and even I began having them myself eight years ago. I have coarse, dead-straight hair, and since I like it to have some shape and direction, a perm is the answer for me. Incidentally, I recommend permanents for men because they give fullness and manageability, especially for men who wash their hair often. And, of course, the same holds true for women.

Recent developments in permanents are perhaps the most exciting innovation in hair care, and used in combination with a good haircut, imagination and good technical knowledge, these permanents can do more to solve hair problems than anything else we've seen in the past decade.

Basically, there are five different types of permanents. I have categorized them by the degree of curl they give to the hair. The degree of curl or wave is controlled by the processing time and the diameter of the rods or rollers which the hair is wrapped on. The smaller the roller, the tighter or frizzier the curl.

1. The strongest kind of permanent will make hair very frizzy. This type of perm was popular in the early seventies. As we made more and more advances with rolling, setting patterns and chemical solutions, this type of perm lost its popularity.

2. Next is a perm that will make small, tight curls ranging from ½ inch to 1 inch in diameter.

3. Wavy perms are perhaps the most popular today. They give loose largish waves from 1½ inches to 2 inches in diameter.

4. A body wave is the mildest permanent. It gives only fullness, and the degree of wave is at most half a curl.

5. A fifth type of permanent is really a permanent in reverse. The chemical solutions are used to straighten very curly or kinky hair.

Permanents and your hair type

Usually I don't recommend a permanent for women with curly or wavy hair. However, if a client has irregular waves or not enough wave or not enough bulk or volume to her hair, I sometimes recommend a permanent to change the direction of the wave, to change the texture, to give more body and/or to make the hair a little more curly. Normally, fine and thin hair takes more time to process. Paradoxically, coarse hair takes a permanent very quickly, so the processing time is quite short. If you have tinted or bleached hair, you must be careful. More about this in the next few pages.

What about home permanents?

I don't recommend permanents to be given at home because if you don't have equal tension and equal amounts of hair on the rods, the results will be uneven, and it's difficult to roll your own hair with the same amount of hair and the same degree of tension on each rod. Also, it's very easy for a novice to bend the

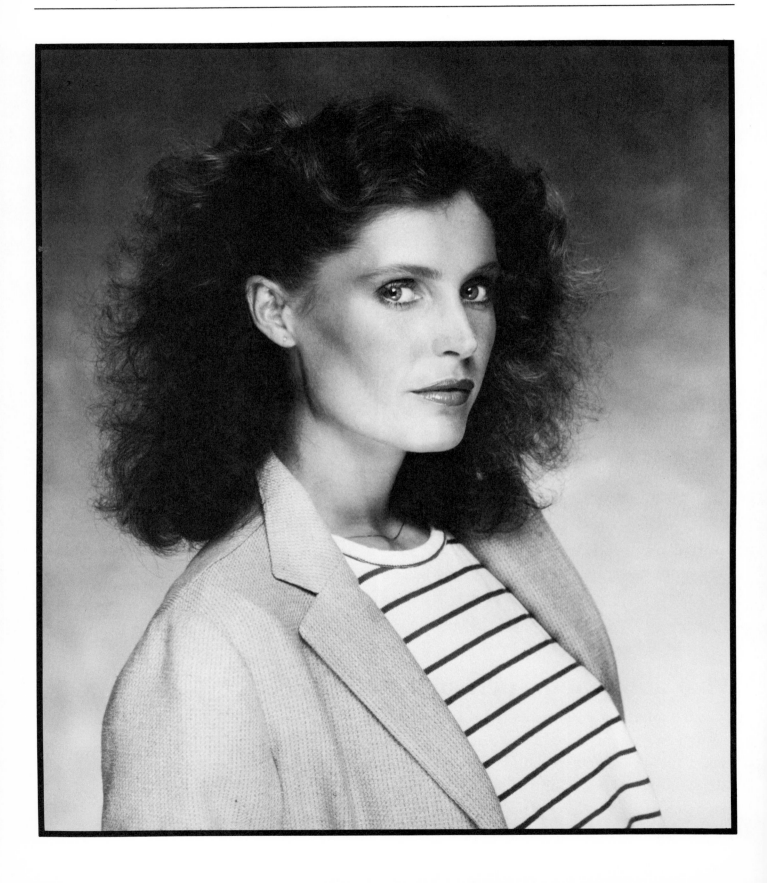

ends of the hair on the rods, and this will leave a permanent and unsightly crimp. The elastic bands that secure the rods can also be placed too tightly and these will give a crimp mark—also permanent. The site of the crimp mark is the place where the hair can easily break, and since this is close to the root, hair breakage at this point can really cause a tragedy. Even if a friend rolls your hair, it's usually no better than doing it yourself because the friend doesn't have the expertise necessary to give the right results.

Can anything be done if a permanent is too strong?

Yes, a permanent can be loosened but it should be done only by a professional. Tell your hairdresser as soon as possible that you are unhappy with your permanent, preferably on the day that you have had it. There is a special technique of combing through the hair to straighten and loosen the perm. The same chemical solutions that were used to curl the hair are used in the combing method. This can be done up to a week after the permanent, but let the salon know as soon as possible that you want it done so you will not be charged for a second perm.

When a permanent is too loose

Wait at least one week and go back to the salon to have it redone. Again, let the salon know as soon as possible that you are dissatisfied with the degree of curl so that you will not be charged for a second perm.

Permanents on tinted, or colored, hair

Today permanents are very definitely possible on tinted hair; in fact, almost any degree of curl is acceptable unless the hair is

Left: This is a permanent with degree #2 of wave. The curls are small and fairly tight and range from ½ to 1 inch in diameter. Good for fine, limp hair.

brittle or damaged. We use milder solutions for colored hair. However, there are a few things to remember: do not have color done for at least two or three weeks before a perm because the process dries the hair. It's wise to condition heavily two to three times before you have the permanent. After you've had the perm, don't panic if the hair goes one or two shades lighter—the chemical solutions tend to strip tinted hair slightly—but the next time you have your hair tinted, the color will be the same as always. You can have your hair tinted a week after the permanent, but condition often and use a mild shampoo.

What about perms on bleached or frosted hair?

This is the most difficult type of hair to permanent because the stripping or bleaching process makes the hair weak and dry, and the results of a permanent on such hair are quite unpredictable. Until a few years ago I never recommended a perm for bleached or frosted hair, but now there are new chemical solutions which are much more gentle and much safer to use than before. The processing for this kind of permanent takes longer, though, so count on spending more time than usual in the salon.

If you have bleached or frosted hair, you need to condition *before* you have a permanent. Use an instant conditioner after each shampoo for the two weeks before the perm. During the same two weeks, use a heavy or penetrating conditioner twice. On the day before you have the permanent, shampoo your hair and give yourself a third penetrating conditioner treatment.

Because I'm so insistent on good conditioning with this type of hair, I often leave an instant conditioner on the hair while I am giving the permanent, or I will sometimes—if the hair appears to be very fragile—mix instant conditioner with the chemical solutions so that the hair is even more protected.

Right: This is a permanent with degree #3 of wave. This is the most popular and versatile perm because it can air-dry naturally, take a set, or be blow-dried.

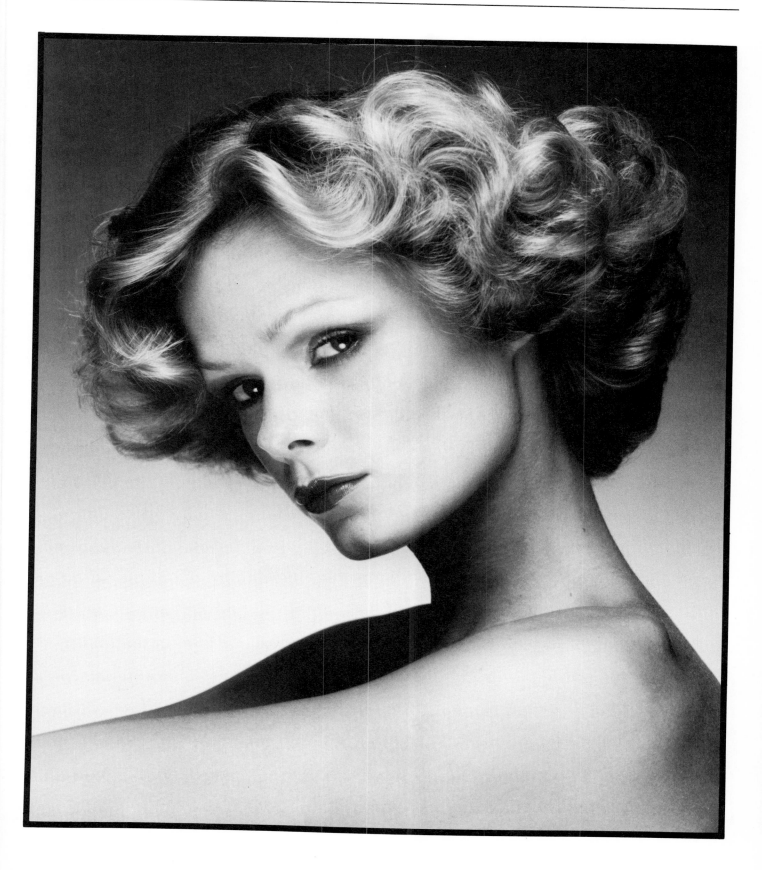

Permanents on hair that has been hennaed or has semipermanent hair coloring

We consider this type of hair somewhere between normal and tinted. But be aware that a permanent will sometimes change the color of the henna and may even remove semipermanent coloring. Wait to have color done two to three days to a week after a perm and be generous with conditioners, using the instant type for the first four shampoos after the perm and then using a heavy conditioner at least once every ten days.

Special precautions about shampooing and conditioning after a perm

After a perm you should wait for two or three days to wash your hair because the shampoo chemicals can loosen the permanent, and the hair needs a rest. If you like to shampoo your hair every day, you can keep doing it, but please, give the hair one day after the perm before washing, and make sure to condition it well.

I do recommend using some kind of instant conditioner for the first four shampoos and then treating the hair once every seven to ten days with a richer creamy or oil-based penetrating conditioner.

I cannot be specific about which shampoo to use because there are so many on the market and each person reacts differently to different shampoos. I can only say you should stay away from strong detergent shampoos if you have a permanent and stick with mild pH-balanced or baby shampoo. I myself have found, after a great deal of experimentation, that a shampoo for tinted hair gives me the most shine, even though my hair is not colored and I only have a mild body perm. When I use a very rich and

Right: Body perm for straight hair gives volume, slight bend. Here, it's blow-dried.

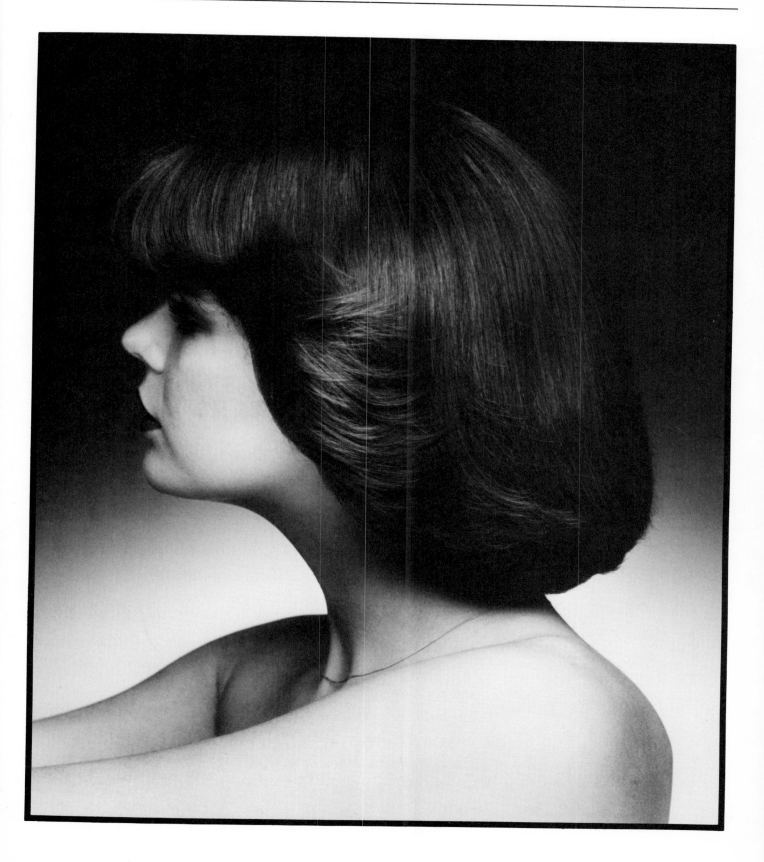

expensive shampoo my hair tends to get greasy; when it is too strong my hair gets dull. So the best course is to keep changing shampoos until you find something that works for you.

When to have a permanent

I feel that the minimum amount of time between permanents is two months. Often a perm will last six months, and the average is about three to four months. Some people don't mind hair that is straight at the roots and curlier at the end, so they wait much longer between perms. Others like the hair near the roots to be curled for height and style; these people will be on the shorter end of the time spectrum between perms. Body perms have to be done most often, about every two or three months because they have the loosest curl.

Partial permanents

When only part of the head is covered with permanent rods or rollers, this is known as a partial permanent. There are many problems that partial perms can solve.

For people who have wavy or curly hair but in one area of the head the hair is straighter than the rest, we'll do a partial perm on that area so the degree of curl will match the rest of the head.

We can also change the direction of the hair. For example, if your hair is short and normally goes downward at the nape of the neck, we can sweep the sides and back upward to give it a new line. This perm is done around the sides only; the crown is left alone. Conversely, you may want height on top of the head, and by combining the right cut with a partial perm, we can give lift and height in the crown area only. Perming at the crown is most successful on short to medium-length hair. If you like a smooth turned-under look, you can have a body wave on the ends of the hair.

Right: Ritsuko has her straight, coarse hair done in a braided permanent (p. 138).

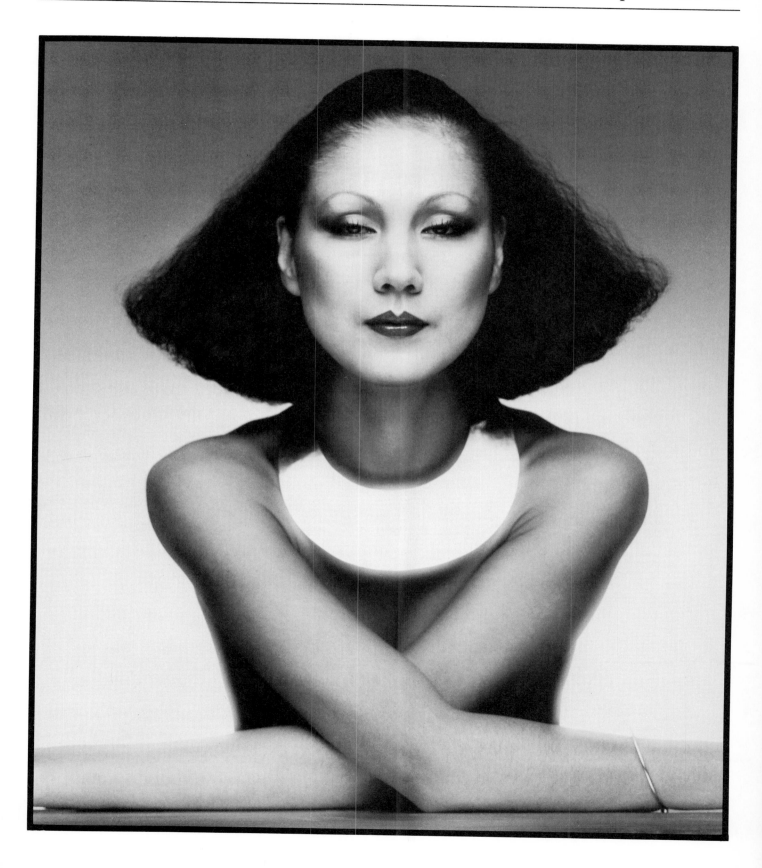

We can also perm just the underlayers of medium- to long-length hair to give more lift and volume. The top layer stays straight and smooth.

Braided permanents

For a Cleopatra look, you can braid the hair in small braids all over the head and apply permanent solutions to the braids. This gives soft, even waves and you must blow-dry or brush-dry to get the proper Egyptian effect. With a Cleopatra style, make sure to have a cut *after* the perm so that the ends are perfectly straight.

Pin-curl permanents

We set hair in pin curls around the face and neck and then apply the solutions. This gives a flat effect and specific direction to the wave of the hair. The crown is set as in a traditional perm on rollers or rods.

For the pin curls, we use a clip made of plastic rather than metal because metal clips cause a negative chemical reaction with the permanent solutions.

Chopstick permanents

For this type of perm, you use a round chopstick-like long rod, measuring about ten inches and made of wood. This kind of perm is specifically for unlayered hair, shoulder-length or longer. It gives an even wave from the root to the ends of hair because the hair is rolled over the complete length of the rod and does not overlap itself. The effect is quite different from a braided perm because the waves are very small and totally even throughout the length of the hair.

Things to remember:

■ If you have medium to long hair, after you have a perm your hair will shorten about 1 to 2 inches because there is more curl to it.

■ Make sure to cover permed hair if you go out in the sun or are exposed to salt water.

■ Even if your hair is "normal" or uncolored, it may lighten a shade or two after a perm.

■ If you have flattened a part of your perm by sleeping on it, you can revive it by misting it with water if you don't feel like washing and drying it.

■ If you have set your permanent or blown it dry to make it straighter or to change the style, don't forget that rain and/or humidity will re-curl it.

■ After a permanent, your hair may have a slight chemical odor if it gets wet. This will go away as soon as it is shampooed and dried. If you cannot wash it, spray some cologne or perfume on your hair to mask the slight chemical smell.

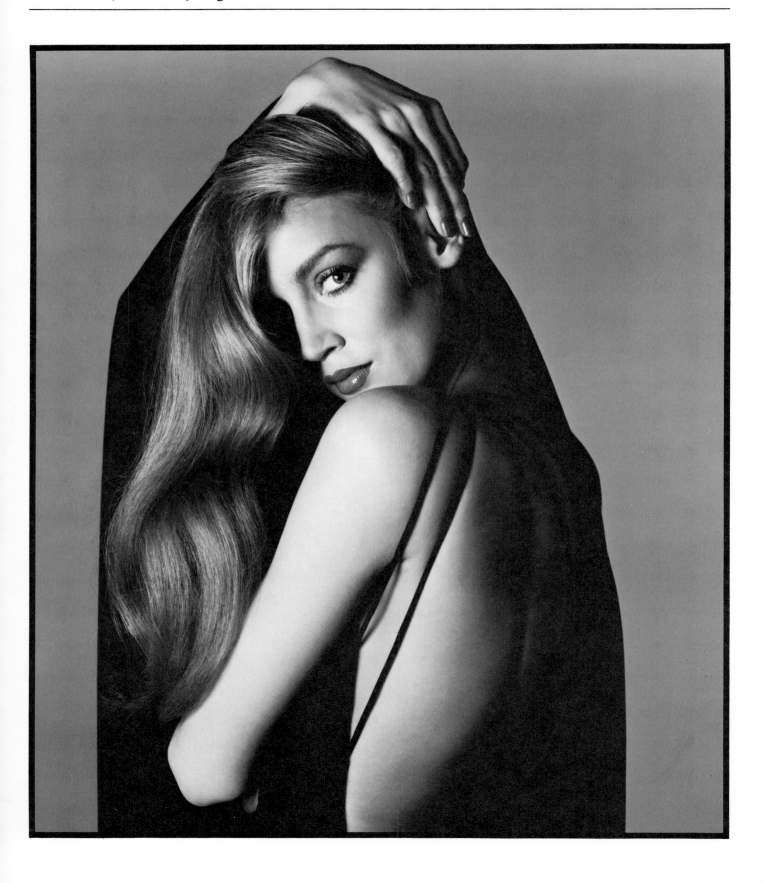

13

What it takes to make your hair look its best: conditioning and care

"Which shampoo should I use?" is the question I am most often asked and every time I have difficulty answering it—for two reasons. First, there are so many shampoos on the market and there is simply no way that I can try all of them, and second, every person's hair reacts differently to different shampoos. However, I can say a few general things about shampoos as they relate to different hair types.

Knowing when, where and how to condition hair is very important. Some hair needs no conditioners, but long, long hair like Jerry Hall's (left) does. Photo, courtesy of Mme. Grès. Photographer: Avedon.

Shampooing normal hair

Some shampoos labeled "For Normal Hair" are strong and overly alkaline. If after using a shampoo twice you find that it makes the hair lose its shine or the scalp or hair itself becomes dry or that the hair becomes dusty or dirty in a day, it is probably because of its strength and/or alkalinity. I usually recommend that you look for a shampoo that is labeled "pH balanced for Normal Hair."

I have also found that very often expensive shampoos or those containing conditioners sometimes have the same dulling and drying effects on the hair. Even if you have normal hair, you might try using shampoos that are labeled "For Tinted Hair" or "For Colored Hair" because they are milder and you may get more shine. But there really is no way of knowing what the best shampoo is until you have experimented and found one that leaves your hair shiny and manageable.

Normal hair should be washed every two to five days but in the summer you probably will want to shampoo it every day or every other day. During warm weather, exposure to sun and salt or chlorinated water makes the hair tend to dryness, so use even a milder shampoo than in the winter months. In general, I'd advise two soapings; the first should be very light and rinsed off right away, and for the second soaping, make a rich lather and massage your scalp with your fingers before you rinse very well.

Shampooing oily hair

If you have oily hair that has not been colored, bleached or has a perm, you should probably use a detergent-type shampoo. Most shampoos designated "For Oily Hair" are detergent-based to cut the soil residue. The best way to recognize whether a shampoo is a detergent or not is the amount of lather that it makes. If you have a rich, very sudsy lather, it's safe to say it's a detergent-based shampoo and to give yourself one or two latherings. If you find that the shampoo is too drying for your hair, use one that's labeled "For Normal Hair" and give yourself two latherings.

If your hair is oily, you must wash often, at the very least once every three days. If it's quite oily or very oily, once a day is what I highly recommend, and give it one lathering only. In the summer all degrees of oily hair should be washed every day—again, lathering the hair only once. If your hair is very oily and you shampoo at night, it may become oily and lose its body and volume by the time you wake up, so I suggest that you wash your hair in the morning if it's possible.

Shampooing dry hair

With dry hair you should definitely use a mild shampoo, perhaps a baby shampoo. If your hair has been full of lotion, grime, spray or conditioners, give it a first soaping with a shampoo for normal hair. The second soaping should always be a shampoo labeled "For Dry Hair." Two lathers is the general rule, but in summer if you are washing more often you should stick to one soaping with a mild or "For Dry Hair" shampoo.

Shampooing combination dry hair and oily scalp

The combination of dry hair and oily scalp is not a condition you're born with. It occurs when you are normally an oily-hair type but have strongly bleached or tinted hair or hair that has been overly processed with chemicals as in perms or straightening. I would suggest a mild shampoo labeled "For Dry Hair," and give yourself two latherings, massaging the shampoo into the scalp and gently soaping the hair itself. You should probably wash this type of hair about every three to five days.

Shampoo tips

The most important thing about a shampoo is the rinsing. Most people don't rinse nearly long enough. Rinse with water that is at a comfortable temperature. After all the suds are out, rinse for at least three minutes and preferably five minutes or more. If you are in a shower, keep your chin down first to rinse, then reverse and keep your chin up so that the whole head is rinsed thoroughly.

Many times I suggest using the coldest tap water as a final rinse for a half minute or so. This closes the pores of the scalp and somehow—I don't know why—for some people this gives a great deal of extra shine and gloss.

Rinses

A rinse is a creamy or watery substance that is applied after shampooing while the hair is still wet. (Color rinses are discussed in the next chapter.) A rinse can accomplish one of several things: it can help to add a little body, it can untangle hair that is difficult to comb or it can add shine.

For *normal hair* you don't need to use a rinse unless your hair tangles very badly; just shampoo and give your hair a thorough water rinse as I've described above.

If you have *oily hair,* you should use an acid-type rinse to give your hair more shine. The creamy-type rinses will only make your hair dirty faster because they are adding more oil where you need less. Here are the recipes I find most effective, which you can easily make yourself:

One pint water to juice of ½ squeezed lemon
or
One pint water to one cup of vinegar

Rinse with either one and leave it in the hair. Vinegar will smell until the hair is dry, but the smell goes away as soon as all the dampness is gone.

If you have *dry hair* or tangled hair, you might try a cream rinse. You should be aware, though, that when you use a cream rinse you lose body, so I generally only recommend rinsing if the hair is especially dry or overly bleached or if it tangles very easily. You must rinse with water even more than usual if you use a cream rinse because the residue can make the hair greasy. One other trick that I've found useful is to mix a teaspoon or two of cream rinse with shampoo when you are doing a second lathering. Make sure your rinsing here is extra long too.

Conditioners

The hair is fed from the scalp; therefore it is necessary to maintain a balanced diet to keep hair healthy. Good sleep and the proper amount of exercise are also necessary to get shiny, glossy, luxurious hair. I know you've heard that a hundred times, but it's really true! In addition to nutrition, rest and exercise, the use of conditioners can help keep your hair supple and shiny. They can also aid in counteracting damage that has been done to hair by bleaches, dyes or permanents.

There are basically two types of conditioners: *penetrating* (sometimes I refer to this kind as a "heavy conditioner") and *instant*. Penetrating conditioners come in rich cream or oily formulations, are usually applied when the hair is clean and should be left on anywhere from twenty minutes to about an hour. The penetrating conditioners penetrate the hair shaft, and replace oils and nutrients that have been lost because of permanents or coloring or overexposure to sun and chlorine. After using a penetrating conditioner, you should wash your hair and dry or set it as usual.

There is a wide variety of heavy conditioners on the market, and the display in your local drugstore can lead to bewilderment about what choice to make. I've found that many brands work well. I've used Clairol's Condition and also the Redken products, which are labeled clearly according to hair type. If you are out of conditioner, you can apply an oil-based product like Elizabeth Arden's 8 Hour Cream to the hair or simply comb baby oil through it and leave on for twenty minutes or more, then shampoo again and rinse *thoroughly.*

The instant conditioners are usually applied after you shampoo. They coat the hair shaft rather than penetrate it and should stay on the hair anywhere from a minute to ten minutes. I've found that Fermodyl's conditioning product labeled "Special" seems to work for most types of hair. Climatress is another instant conditioner that's widely available in drugstores.

After the allotted time on the hair, most instant conditioners should be rinsed off with water; a few should be left on the hair while you go on with setting and drying as usual. As I said, instant conditioners coat the hair shaft with softeners and nutrients, but the effects of the conditioners will wash out with your next shampoo.

There are times when the hair simply won't respond to conditioners of any kind. When you are sick, even with an ordinary head cold, your hair will not shine as much and conditioners probably won't help, so you'll just have to wait until you get better. Tension and nervousness can affect hair too and sometimes may even cause spotty baldness. If loss of hair is from stress and nervousness, it will usually grow back, but in any case, see a dermatologist right away.

If hair is severely damaged by overbleaching, overprocessed permanents or if it is burnt, conditioners will not do very much for it. The only way to healthy hair is to let it grow. I usually suggest to a client who has badly damaged hair that she cut it as short as possible so that the new growth is healthy. If she doesn't want to cut her hair, then the only alternative is to wait until it grows to a manageable or attractive length and then cut off the damaged portion.

Any strong medication, especially hormones, cortisone and birth-control pills, may have adverse effects on hair. When you have problem hair or are losing your hair, the best and safest thing to do is to go to a dermatologist to find out what is causing the problems. We hairdressers can condition the hair, but we cannot cure the causes of hair problems. In addition, remember that when you worry about hair problems they get even worse, so go quickly to a doctor to avoid multiplying your problems.

Conditioning for normal hair

If you have virgin hair (meaning hair that has not been colored, bleached, tinted, hennaed or permanented), then I don't feel it's necessary to use a conditioner. If you have any one of the above and you feel your hair is still in the category of "normal," I recommend the instant conditioners. If your hair is tinted or permed, use an instant conditioner each time you wash for two or three weeks following the coloring or permanent, and thereafter use every other time you shampoo.

Conditioning for oily hair

You really don't have to use a conditioner because your kind of hair is supplied with an abundance of its own natural oils. If you want more shine, use the vinegar rinse recommended under "Rinses" (above).

Conditioning for dry hair

Use an instant conditioner every time you wash your hair, and use a heavy or so-called penetrating conditioner once every ten days. In summer when your hair is extra dry and you are in direct sunlight, comb rich conditioner or baby oil directly into your hair and go to the beach or sit by the pool with your hair slicked back or tied into a knot. After you come in from the sun your hair may have caked or dried, but it will have been fully protected and given a conditioning treatment at the same time. You must shampoo the hair very, very well, three or more soapings should dislodge any caked-on conditioner or oil—and of course, use a mild shampoo or baby shampoo.

Conditioning for tinted, permed or bleached hair

Use an instant conditioner every time you shampoo for the first two or three weeks after your hair has been chemically treated. Then use a heavy or penetrating conditioner once every two weeks, leaving it on the hair for at least thirty minutes.

After shampooing, apply the heavy conditioner and massage it into the hair and scalp. Comb the conditioner evenly through your hair, then put a snug plastic bag over your hair and leave the bag on for thirty minutes at least (an hour is preferable). If you have a heating cap, over-the-head dryer or heat lamp, stay under it (with the plastic bag on) for thirty minutes—the hot air helps the conditioner to work better. Wash your hair two or three times until no trace of conditioner is left and rinse with water extra thoroughly—five minutes at least.

Continue this routine the year round, but in the summer you may want to deep-condition more often. Try to keep your hair covered with a scarf or hat at all times if you are in the sun for any length of time.

Conditioning for dry scalp or mild dandruff

If you have either of these conditions, I suggest you try an oil treatment once a week especially in winter, when there is less moisture in the air and the hair gets even drier.

Section your hair into four layers starting from a center part, and thoroughly saturate the hair with baby or castor oil. Use cotton balls or cotton pads and make sure every strand of hair is heavily coated. Then massage the scalp, put on a snug-fitting plastic bag and leave it on for at least an hour. If you want to speed up the process, sit under a dryer for a half-hour to forty-five minutes. I have heard that oil treatments can very slightly lift the color from processed or colored hair, but I have seen no evidence to support this and I have always found oil treatments to be safe and effective.

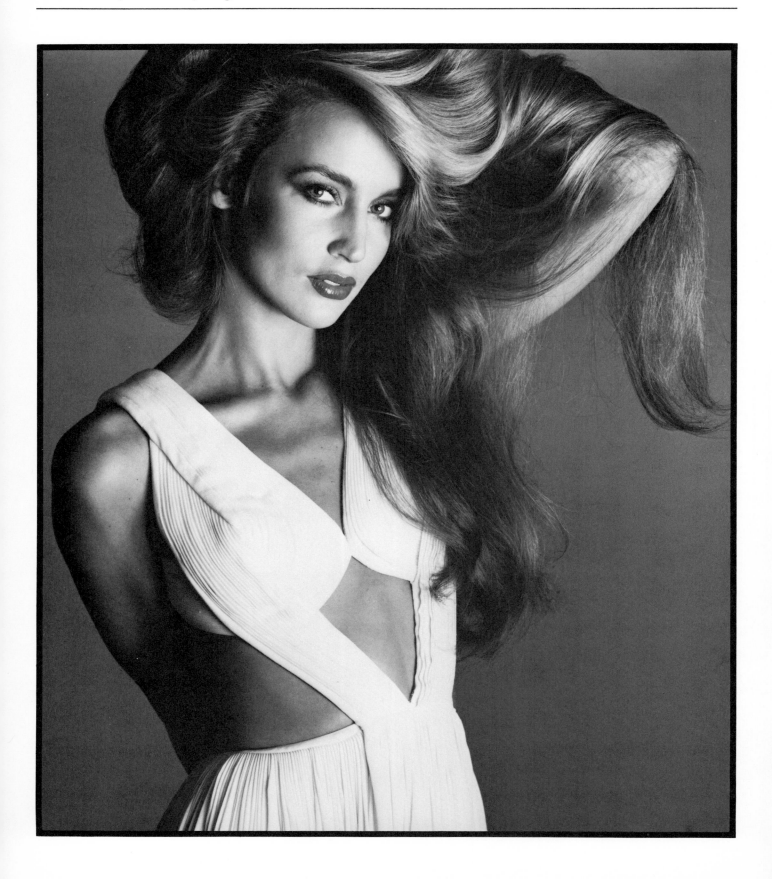

14

Hair coloring: a natural approach

There are really only two good reasons to use hair coloring. One is to change the color of your hair to achieve a different look, and the other is to cover gray. Seventy percent or more of my clients use color on their hair. Today we have many inventive methods of hair coloring: hair painting, streaking and sunbursting are common now, but combinations of semipermanent color and henna rinses are newer, and much interesting work with this kind of color is being done in salons in large cities across the country.

Left: Hair coloring and highlighting should look as natural as possible. Photo, courtesy of Mme. Grès. Photographer: Avedon.

Finding a good colorist is crucially important. I'm always interested in the kind of background experience colorists come to me with. Many have worked in the labs of the large commercial hair-coloring manufacturers; others have trained in salons under master colorists. A colorist must have an aesthetic sense: I mean, he or she must be able to mix and use color to make a natural look. Anything artificial with hair color is very unattractive, at least to my eyes. When you look for a colorist, the best rule to follow is to look at the work he is doing in the salon. No use stopping someone in the street and asking her where she had her color done—it's obviously artificial-looking if you can spot it enough to ask where it was done. There are now salons which specialize only in color. They may be fine, but don't forget that a good colorist is like a good stylist: he may not be in the most expensive or chic salon—it's the quality of the work that counts.

As a general guideline about coloring, I do not like to suggest anything lighter or darker than two shades different from your own natural color. Gray hair is an exception, and I'll talk about that later.

Your skin tone is the most important factor in choosing hair color. Olive skin almost never looks natural with very blond hair, nor does it look right with overly reddish hair. Conversely, very fair skin may look too washed-out with blond hair or too pale with hair that's very dark.

The color of your eyebrows must of course relate to the color you choose—another reason not to go more than two shades lighter or darker than what you were born with.

I sometimes like to see hair brightened up, adding a bit of highlight to the natural color. The effect should be as if the sun is touching your hair. If you are considering this kind of highlighting, streaking or sunbursting, please remember that even highlights shouldn't go more than two shades lighter, or they too will look artificial.

Lighter brown or medium and darker brown hair streaking can look interesting on many skin colors, but beware of too much redness. Since brunettes sometimes have a great deal of red in their hair pigmentation, they run the risk of reddish streaks in the highlighting process which can often look too harsh. Stay away from this unless you like the effect and it works well with your skin color.

If you have brown hair and discover reddish or brassy streaks after the highlighting process, you can always tone them down with a temporary rinse that mutes the color or you can cover the whole head with semipermanent color until it grows out.

When you go more than two shades different from your own natural color you probably have to have color done every three to four weeks and this is too much—too much damage to the hair, too much time and too much money. Even if you color only the new growth, it is impossible not to overlap the chemicals onto the hair that has already been colored. This immediately overdries the hair and makes it susceptible to breakage.

I am really against what is known as two-process coloring, which means stripping or bleaching the hair (the first process) before adding the coloring (the second process). The reasons for this are quite simple. As I said, I am against unnatural hair color, and if you have to strip or bleach the hair of its natural color, the result will inevitably be hair that is more than two shades lighter than before. Two-process coloring is also one of the leading causes of damage to the hair because the harsh chemicals used to bleach the hair weaken it greatly and can cause severe breakage.

Some new thoughts on gray hair

When I see a woman with a head of beautiful gray or white hair I often think of her as intelligent and classy, as was the late Mrs. William Paley. Many women who color their gray should let it go natural; it can look amazingly beautiful and very sophisticated.

But in some cases when a client asks, "Should I go gray?," I say no when I think she would look older instead of better.

But I have often seen women who have been coloring their hair and then decide to let it go fully gray or white look years younger with the softness of natural gray. Other women may need color around their face, or the gray that they have is not quite gray enough, and to these I suggest a very natural hair coloring.

When you have just a little gray in an otherwise dark head of hair, you will notice it more quickly because of the contrast. Once you are obviously getting gray you should decide if you want to let it grow naturally or color your hair.

If you are turning gray and you have lighter hair, you might decide to add highlights or paint in some lighter streaks to blend in with the white hairs. The effect will be a mix of natural color plus gray plus added color, and all this adds up to a very attractive look.

If you want to go gray, there is usually a period when you get an uneven salt-and-pepper look which can be annoying. This is the time to use temporary or a semipermanent rinse. If you have put permanent color over gray and you decide you want to let it grow naturally, I would suggest that you put semipermanent color on the roots only. However, this will never color the white as much as permanent color and you will probably be uncomfortable with this look, but you have to go through it to get what you want. I'd suggest that at this time you cut your hair short, in a layered cut. Hair color shows more in smooth and straight hair; if the hair is more tousled and curled, the color is less obvious. I never recommend that gray hair be longer than chin length, anyway, because it tends to age you unless you're going to wear it tied back into a chignon or knot.

Sometimes new gray hair has a different texture from your regular hair. The new gray hair may be more wiry or more curly. (If this bothers you, don't pull out the offending hairs, because if you do, you'll have less hair in the future.) I'm often asked if the texture of hair all over the head will change as the hair turns gray. I cannot predict about the texture of hair based only on the first gray hairs. You must wait at least until a third or fourth of the total hair is gray. Usually the degree in difference between your natural hair and the gray seems more dramatic at first, but after it's totally gray it's probably not going to be that drastically different in texture.

You cannot make gray hair completely white. You cannot bleach gray hair to white because it has no pigment. (However, gray hair will take permanent color.) If you are over 80 percent gray, you cannot frost or streak, since the bleach will not take, so you must color it darker or decide to let it go completely natural.

Permanent hair coloring

Permanent color is any hair dye which permanently changes the hair color. The solutions for permanent hair coloring usually contain peroxide, which changes the natural structure of the hair. Permanent color can sometimes cause the hair texture to become coarser and drier. Quite often you will find that your hair tangles more easily and is harder to comb after the permanent-color process.

Semipermanent hair color

Semipermanent color does not contain peroxide and therefore does not change the structure or the texture of the hair. You can think of it as coating but not penetrating the hair the way permanent color does. However, if you apply semipermanent hair coloring often enough (every two or three weeks), it can change the color of your hair permanently. There is more color on darker hair tones from repeated applications. I like using semipermanent color especially on dark hair, as it gives a rich deep color without changing the texture or overly drying the hair.

Semipermanent color processing can be done at home but it tends to be quite messy. I prefer the foam type product, as it is easier to control—you can leave it on the hair longer and go about your work, since it does not run onto to your clothes as easily as the liquid products. If you want to cover gray, I would suggest leaving the foam on about double the time that the directions indicate. Usually the process should be repeated about every five to six weeks, but you can repeat up to every other week. Remember, the more often you apply semipermanent color, the more the hair is coated with color and the degree of color becomes permanent after a while. If you eventually want to go gray or fully natural, you cannot repeat the coloring process more than every five to six weeks because the hair shaft becomes permanently coated with color and will not wash out.

Quite often semipermanent rinses give a great deal of shine to the hair. Each head of hair is different and there's really no way of predicting who will have more shine and who won't. Also, don't forget that some of the semipermanent color will wash out in every shampoo, so your suds and water may be lightly colored. If you wash your hair every day, semipermanent color will wash out in about two to three weeks unless you have built up the color by repeated applications. Always use a very mild shampoo so that there is as little stripping or fading of color as possible.

Temporary color

Temporary color really does not color the hair, it just gives it tone. Usually it is to be used just after shampooing and towel-drying. It works best on slightly damp hair and will not change the hair more than one shade at most. If you want to be a little redder or a little grayer or kill yellow in gray hair, this is a good but very temporary way to do it, as this kind of rinse comes out in one wash. If you use temporary rinses too often they can stain your pillowcases, and even your collars if you have long hair.

Henna

Henna is probably the healthiest color processing you can use. It is historically the oldest method of hair coloring. It is completely organic and comes in a powdery form with a smell faintly reminiscent of hay. Henna, like semipermanent color, coats the hair shaft but does not penetrate it. Because of the coating action, henna tends to give the hair a bit more body and shine. Red henna has become increasingly fashionable in the last few years, but there are two other true colors in henna—black and brown. There is also a non-color known as natural henna. The three shades can be mixed, but there is not as much subtlety in the color range as in the synthetic commercial products that are most widely used in salons and at home.

One of the major problems with henna is that it reacts differently on different types of hair. It can also take a long time to process, from a half-hour to an hour and even more.

Natural henna gives a shine for certain kinds of hair but sometimes changes the hair color. For example, I have seen blond hair turn to green when natural henna has been used on it. If you are thinking of using natural henna and your hair is a very light shade, I would suggest staying away from it, or at the very least trying a small patch test on some strands of underhair. I often recommend that natural henna be used on darker virgin hair as a revitalizer which gives shine and body.

Henna is stronger than semipermanent color, but not as strong as permanent color. It does not coat gray completely and sometimes I find the effect of orangish blond hairs mixed with darker hair (which is what most often happens when you are coating gray with henna) to be unattractive. Henna does wash out of the hair, but not as quickly as semipermanent coloring. Like semipermanent color it may become permanent if used very often, and if it is used repeatedly without conditioning, it can sometimes overly dry the hair. If you are having a perm, make sure you have your henna done at least a week before.

Bleaching and highlighting

Bleaching removes color from natural hair, but you never know what the end results will be until it's done. In darker hair shades the pigmentation may be heavily red and you may be surprised at the color as the bleaching process takes place. Years ago bleach was used as a first process to strip the color of the hair. Color would then be added to the bleached hair. But today bleach is more widely used as part of a highlighting.

There are many different names given to what is usually called highlighting. Frosting, streaking, sunbursting, painting are just a few in use today. The highlighting process basically consists of bleaching strands of hair for different lengths of time so that they will be bleached in a variety of shades. (The length of time that you leave bleach on the hair is what counts; the longer you leave on the bleach, the lighter the hair becomes.) The effect of this kind of bleaching can be very natural, but this should be done only by professionals because the timing and the types of bleach used make the process very tricky and difficult to do at home.

One other caution about bleaching: Don't try to bleach the hair to white; it will never work. The hair can be bleached out to almost white, but some yellow or red residue will remain. When you bleach, the structure of the hair is changed and it becomes coarser and drier, increasingly brittle and subject to breakage. Therefore it is very important that you condition it well and try to do as little as possible to the hair: don't use hot rollers or electric curling irons too often, and don't have a permanent unless a professional says that your hair can tolerate one. If you're considering a vacation in the sun or it is summertime, have your highlighting done before you go but take into account that the sun and salty air and chlorinated water all tend to strip your hair of color and therefore make it even lighter. Tell your colorist of your vacation plans and he or she will leave the bleach on your hair for less time than usual and the sun will do the rest to make your highlighting the same as it always is.

Tip for men about highlighting

Men who have *light* hair naturally, and find themselves with a receding hairline or thinning hair, might consider highlighting or painting because it makes the hair color closer to the skin color, and baldness becomes less obvious. For men, I recommend that this be done right before summer when the sun will probably help bleach the hair, anyway, and the look is completely natural. This may be done twice a year.

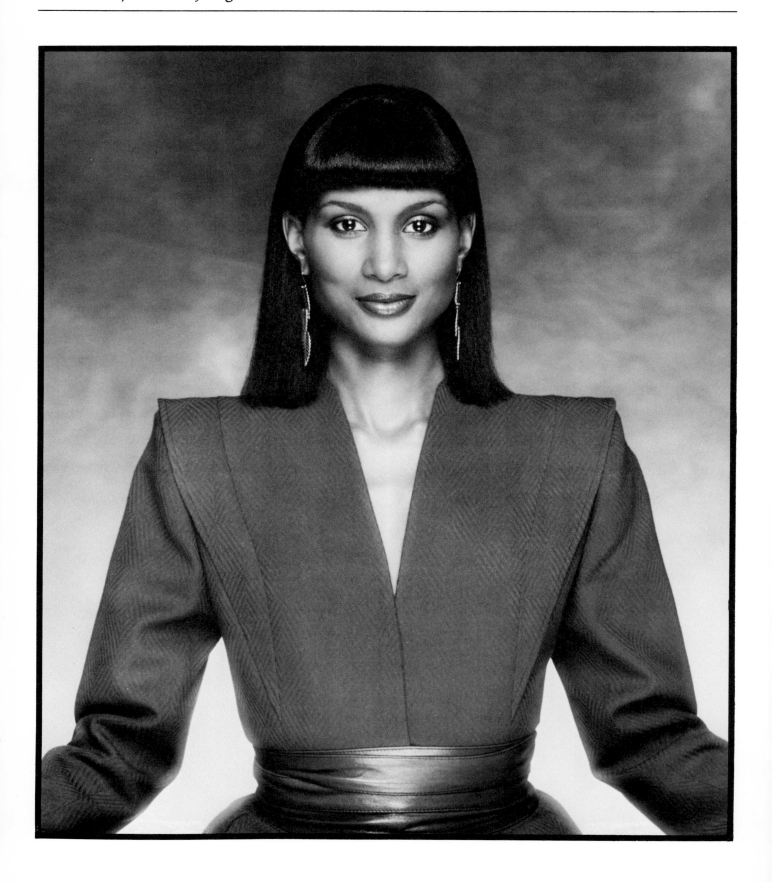

15

A new view on hairpieces

Hairpieces of all kinds have been around at least since Cleopatra's time. When you say "hairpiece" today, many people tend to think of the heavy falls and switches that were very fashionable in the late sixties. These gave an artificial look, and to my mind, today they seem old-fashioned and very unnatural.

Many new little hairpieces have been developed in the last few years. The use of synthetic fibers has made pieces very affordable, and today a woman can buy several small hairpieces that will give her a great deal of versatility.

Left: Small hairpieces can change your look totally. Experiment with bangs, strips or tails.

I don't think a hairpiece should be used to dramatically change your look; it should be used to make a particular look or style better. By that I mean that wearing a blond wig if you have naturally brown hair will be too dramatic, too artificial, but using a small strip or switch of hair to make a perfect French twist or a beautifully rounded chignon makes good sense. Hairpieces can also be used to give fullness to your hair. Little pieces can easily be attached to the crown for volume, and new thin strips of hair made from synthetic fibers can be used to make bangs or give you thick rich bangs when combined with your own hair, or they can be attached to the back of the head below the crown to give you a glamorous look of thick hair. Pieces can be used to make ponytails and chignons, and they can be used as rolls or fillers.

Consult with your hairdresser about which hairpieces would work for you. In addition, go to a good wigmaker and ask to see what new little pieces he has and what he would recommend for you. Once you have purchased a piece, ask your hairdresser to help you use it and to give you some new ideas. Don't plan on wearing your hairpiece until you have had time to practice with it. After two or three practice sessions you should have the knack of exactly where to place it and how to fasten it so that it feels secure.

Wigs are another matter. I feel you can almost always know that a wig is a wig, and therefore the look is unnatural. Of course, if you have a severe problem, a wig is the best solution and I strongly advise consulting a fine wigmaker and spending as much as you can possibly afford to get the highest quality. In case you must wear a wig every day, I recommend natural hair or a combination of natural and synthetic, and if possible, you should buy a wig that allows you to comb the hair around your hairline directly into the wig so that there is a feeling of naturalness about it.

Right: Margaux Hemingway has fine hair, adds a small switch to make a thick braid.

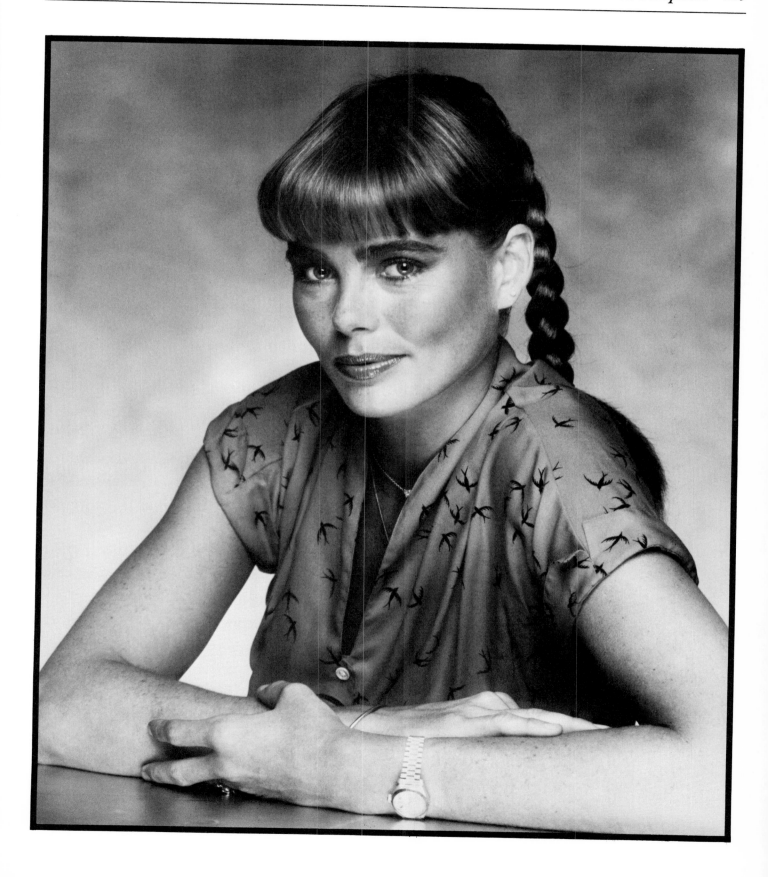

What to look for

The following are some guidelines about what to look for when buying a hairpiece (or a wig):

1. The most important factor in buying a hairpiece is to match the color of your hair.

2. Make sure that your natural hairline shows at some point (probably it will be at the forehead or sides) because it is difficult to detect a piece if your own hair is combed through it or combined with it.

3. The texture of the hair on the piece should match the texture of your own hair (fine, coarse, medium) as closely as possible, and the degree of wave should also be close to that of your own hair.

4. Remember that too much hair looks unreal. The less hair on a piece, the more desirable it is because it gives a much more natural look.

Synthetic or natural?

There are two major differences between hairpieces made of human hair and those made of synthetic fibers. First, human hair tangles much more than synthetic hair and needs far more care and upkeep. Second, synthetic hair is much lighter, easier to wash and dry, and usually does not have to be reset. It is also weatherproof, meaning that it will not lose its curl in humidity and rain as a natural hairpiece does, and it is less expensive.

I most often recommend synthetics when a woman is considering buying a smallish hairpiece. For a larger piece, I sometimes recommend ordering a mix of human hair and synthetic.

You must be careful when purchasing a synthetic piece. Be choosy when it comes to fibers. Most people pick up pieces that are too shiny and don't look natural. The newer ones are less shiny, much closer to the quality of real hair, and depending on

Right: Do you recognize Lauren Hutton? She wears a little-boy wig that was cut on her head so that the shape would be perfectly right. Photo, courtesy of *Vogue*, Condé Nast Publications. Photographer: Avedon.

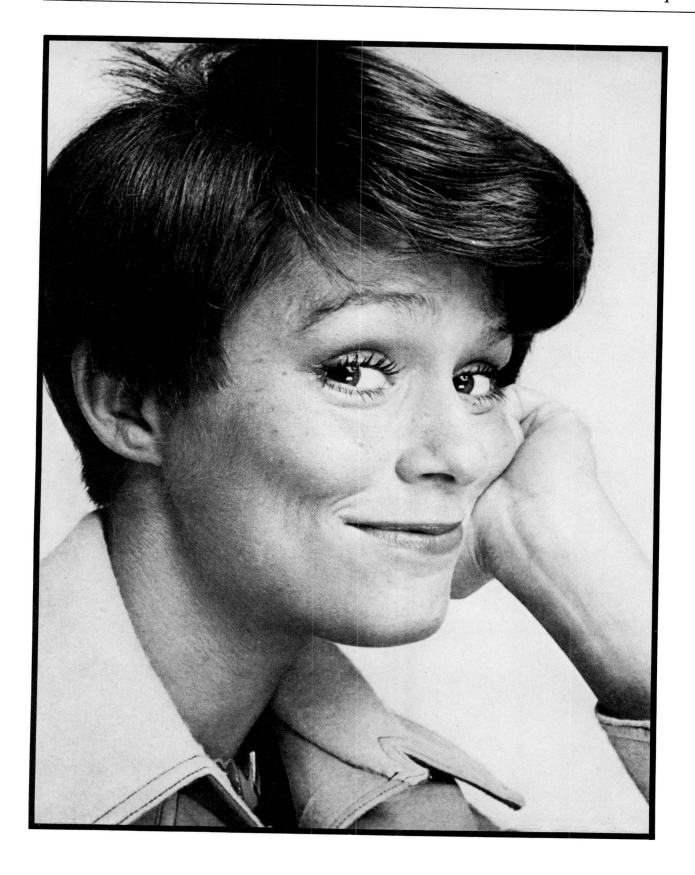

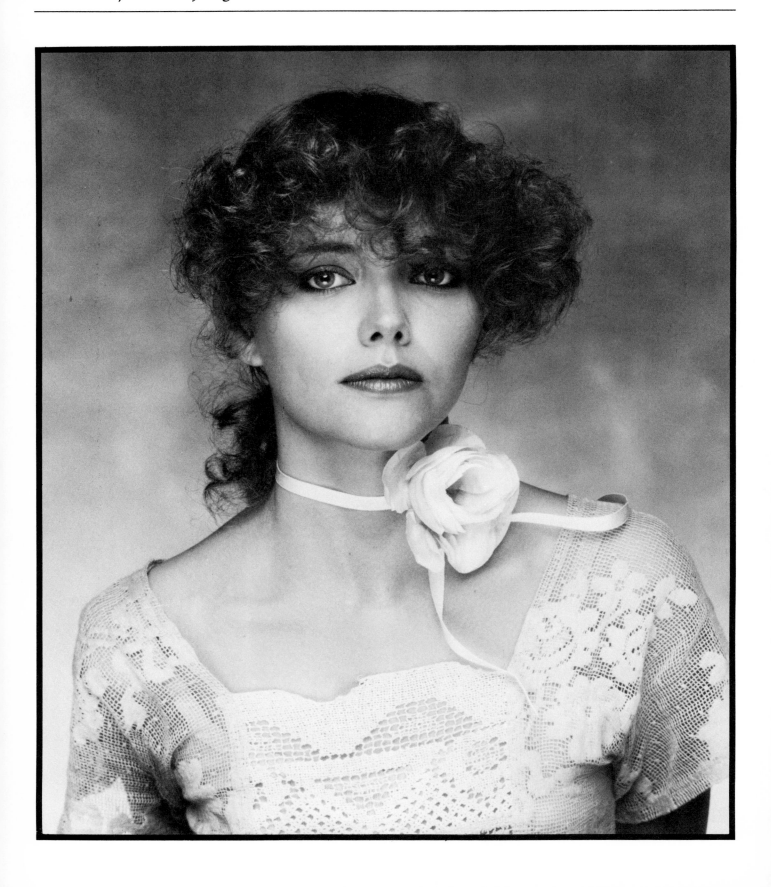

the fiber, they can be reset or not. Before you buy a piece, ask if it is resettable or not. You may want one where the style can be changed or you may prefer the piece to keep its style throughout its life. In any case, they are all easily washable.

The pieces I think are most versatile are:

Long thin strips with permanently set fibers on them. The fibers, or "hair," range from curly to wavy and from about 4 to 10 inches in length. You can buy this type of strip by the yard and cut it to the length that you need. A strip can be used for bangs only, or you can attach it with bobby pins to the back of your head near the back of each ear to give length and fullness. It makes a good "filler" to roll or comb your own hair around, and it can be used to give fullness at the top of the crown or almost anywhere. Strips of different lengths are ideal for traveling or instant changes, and you simply anchor them to your head with bobby pins.

Another kind of highly useful piece is the thin switch, about 18 to 20 inches long. This is the best kind of piece to give fullness to a chignon or to be combined with your own hair to make a plump braid, or it can be used to make twists or rolls. It should

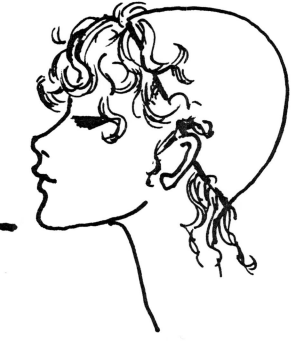

Small strips of synthetic fiber that are sold by the yard are used *(left)* like a headband, to extend the volume of hair. Measure the amount you'll need, simply snip off, attach with bobby pins. (See p. 58 for the same haircut without hairpiece.)
Photo: Skrebneski

be thin—that is, not much hair should be on it—and it can be attached with bobby pins or hairpins.

A piece that I consider most versatile measures from 1 to 1½ inches in width at the base and has hair measuring from 6 to 8 inches in length. This kind is sometimes hard to find but can be ordered from wigmakers. Basically, it is a contemporary version of a fall and attaches with small combs just below the crown of the head. Best use is for someone who has long hair but wants to make it more luxurious by making it a bit fuller.

The "nearly-wig" is what I recommend for women who need or prefer to use a wig. This kind of piece covers 90 percent of the hair, but the natural hair around the face is exposed and brushed into the wig. You could use this to change the length of your hair, or if you travel a great deal and need to have your hair looking good at all times.

If you have a special need or you can't find exactly what you want, you can always design your own piece. For instance, you may want straight China-doll bangs (which are very charming with a ponytail) or a piece that just fits the crown of your head to give you height. You can give your specifications to any fine wigmaker and together you will come up with a piece that can solve your particular needs.

Note: When you are having a hairpiece cut or trimmed, *always* have it done on your head. This applies to even the smallest piece. When you have a piece cut on your head, the stylist can work with your natural hair and the shape of your skull to make it look as natural as possible.

Washing hairpieces

If your hairpiece is synthetic, just brush it first and wash in lukewarm water and Woolite. Don't rub it or twist it; just dip it in and out of soapy water and comb it through gently, and then rinse it well in cool water. Pat it dry with a towel and shake it well, and simply hang it up to dry.

If the piece is human hair or a combination of human hair and synthetics, take it back to where you bought it to have it cleaned and set.

It's very difficult to say how often to wash and/or set a piece. It depends on frequency of use and the conditions under which you are using it. If it's hot and humid, you'll probably want to wash it rather often, just as you would your own hair.

FLYING HAIRPIECES

A few years ago Mme. Hanae Mori was doing her first fashion show in Paris and I was flown over to do the hair. We were all very nervous and I had only one assistant backstage with twelve models to do. When you're backstage at an important fashion show it's a madhouse—the pandemonium back there is totally opposite from what's happening out front.

Each of the models was to have a similar hair style that I had designed for Mme. Mori. It involved a small Japanese samurai knot, or chignon, on the crown of the head.

The music started and the girls all lined up to make their grand entrances when I suddenly noticed that one of the girls looked different—she had no knot. I ran to the front and stuck a chignon on her with one hairpin—I didn't have a bobby pin, which would at least have been stronger. Unfortunately, she had short fine hair, which made the anchoring of the knot even harder. I warned her to be "very careful."

The girls began to go out onstage and do their twirls, and I was peeking behind the curtain when the chignon I had hairpinned flew off the model's head and landed directly by Sophia Loren's left foot.

When the show was finished I thought it was the end of me, too. I apologized to Mme. Mori, expecting the worst. She said, "Oh, it was wonderful because the mood was very tense until the hairpiece came off, and then the show started to come alive." I've been doing the hair for Mme. Mori's shows ever since.

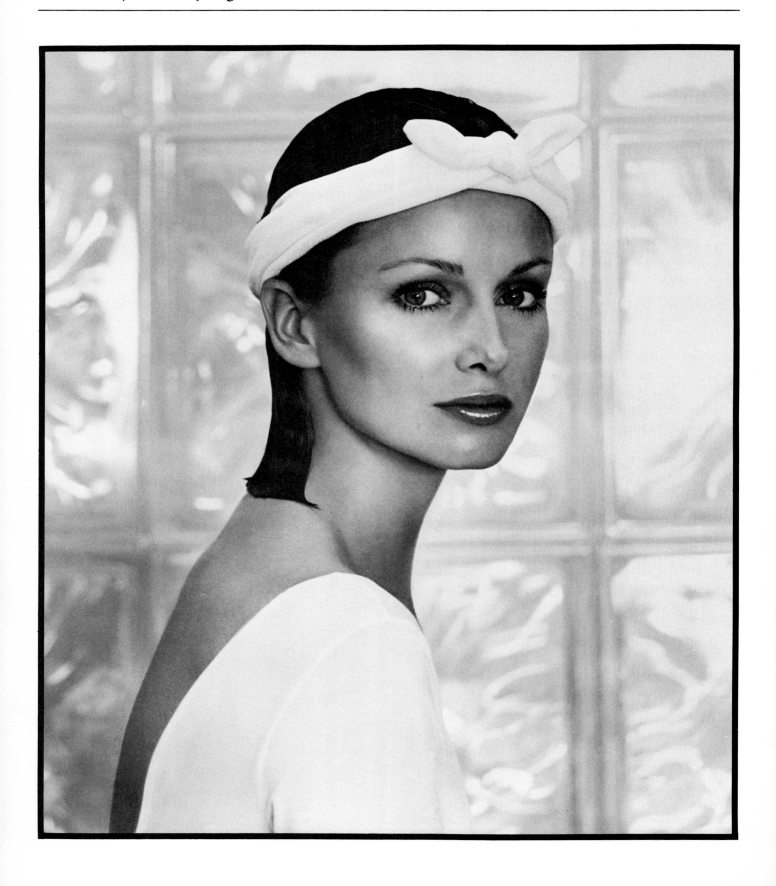

16

Traveling

Traveling presents special problems. It's usually a time when you want to look your best and have the least time. In addition, atmospheric conditions—humidity, rain, dryness, snow—all contribute to making it difficult to handle your hair when you travel. There are a few things that you can do, however, to make your hair and your life bearable when you're on the go.

The first thing I usually advise is that you take whatever you normally use by way of a comb or brush. If you are fond of a very large brush, take it; you'll feel far more comfortable with it, even if it means using a few more cubic inches in your suitcase.

Left: Karen Graham is a world-traveler. When she's on the beach she just slicks her hair back with conditioner, ties it with a chic terry wrap. Photo, courtesy of Estée Lauder. Photographer: Skrebneski.

Then, if you don't already have one, consider buying a less bulky or heavy dryer than you normally use, but remember that it should have enough power to dry the hair quickly and efficiently. A dryer with 800 watts of power or more is what you need to do the job. Depending on where you're going, check on the electrical current (travel agents know about these things) and get an adapter if you need one. If you are staying in a big city, the housekeeper in the hotel can usually supply an adapter, but it's a good idea to bring one. They cost very little and are usually small and lightweight.

If you want to use electric rollers, take the smallest ones you have. Again, if you're traveling in a foreign country, you have to check on the voltage. If you can't take electric rollers, I've found that a handy substitute is to take sponge rollers. They are light, have no bulk and can be pressed into unlikely corners in your suitcase. They can be used for a set after a shampoo and dried with a dryer or left on overnight. Take a size smaller in sponge rollers than you normally would because you'll be leaving them in for a shorter time, and the curl will be tighter if the diameter of the roller is smaller.

If you are stuck without a dryer, here too you might try asking the housekeeper in a large hotel if there are any available. If not, use the finger-comb or brush-dry techniques.

If you are going on a long trip, have your hair cut before you leave. But don't just tell your hairdresser you want it cut "shorter to last for the trip" because you will probably be uncomfortable with it for the first two or three weeks. Ask him what he recommends as the best way to handle your hair. Perhaps this is a good time to consider having a body wave or permanent.

If you go to a foreign city and you need a salon set, try the hotel's beauty salon and explain what set is normally done on your hair. Don't get upset if you don't get the same results; you can always brush it close to the look that you usually have as soon as you get to your room, and there's no major disaster, since you have not had it cut.

When you go to a foreign country, sometimes your shampoo does not work because the water is different. Bring your own shampoo; often it will behave as it does at home, but if it doesn't, buy one of the shampoos made in that country. Remember, with water that is different, the hair must be rinsed even longer than normally—five minutes or more is minimum time.

Note: Small hairpieces can often save the day—or night—so think about buying one before you leave. Buy it so you have plenty of time for experimentation before you take your trip, and tell your hairdresser that you'd like a quick lesson or two on how to use it.

Traveling to a humid climate

The humidity on a Caribbean island or in the tropics will undo any style, so the trick is to go with the weather. Humidity will uncurl a set, or curl or straighten blow-dried hair, and it will always bring out the natural state of the hair, whether curly or straight.

The best attitude to take is not to fret: go with it, or you won't enjoy yourself. I find it incongruous to see a woman on a beach with perfectly coiffed hair. The more natural the look, the more becoming it is on a beach or boat. Combs, barrettes, ribbons and elastic bands are useful extras to bring even if you don't normally use them. Think of using tropical flowers for evening: just pin them in—they'll give any look a little more charm.

When you are on a winter vacation or in the tropics, make-up is probably a more important factor than hair because you have much more control over it and it takes away the emphasis on the hair. Sleeked-back hair (using a setting gel or conditioning lotion or just plain baby oil) with more dramatic eye make-up than you usually wear is a good look for southern or humid climates.

If you simply give up all hope on your hair, a neat scarf or a turban wrap is chic and hides all problems. But as I said, you'll probably be more comfortable if you just let it all hang out. It has always surprised me that so many women are not aware that the stiff, artificial look of every hair in place is really out of place in more relaxed surroundings. Hair that's left to its own devices moves freely and easily and takes a great deal of the burden of worrying about it off you—and it seems to me that that's what vacations are all about.

CRYING IN THE RAIN

I went to Mexico with *Vogue* one September and we didn't know it was the rainy season. The editor on this trip wanted the models' hair to be very curly for each picture. In those days I was using lots of hairpieces, and every night for three weeks I was setting hairpieces on small rollers. Because of the heat we had to start work at five in the morning. This meant that the models got up at three to put on make-up, and I woke up at four to start the hair. Most of the time the morning mist had made their hair straight by the time we got on location.

The editor was so insistent about having the right fashion look for the pictures that she told me to take an old-fashioned curling iron that she had with her and to heat it over an alcohol lamp. Not only that, she wanted me to do it on top of a pyramid where we did most of the shots.

Every day all of us (except the editor) cried at one point or another—the models, the photographer, the photographer's assistant and I. Finally, when the three weeks were up, we were told that we had still more work to do. I secretly called the assistant to the editor in chief of *Vogue* and offered to pay for another hairdresser to come and take my place. I was at Kenneth's at the time and of course risked my job by calling her, but she persuaded me to stay. The moral of this story is that the hair you see in pictures is not necessarily the hair that goes with the climate.

Right: Rolling or twisting when your hair is wet gives a sleek, sophisticated look. If you comb conditioner through wet hair and sit in the sun, your hair is protected and treated at the same time.

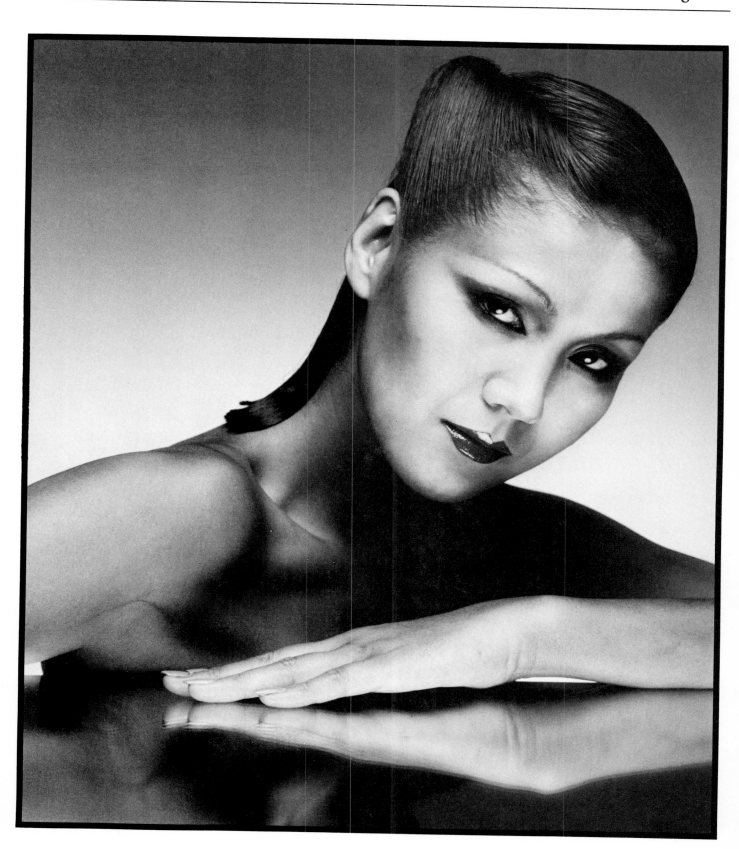

V.I.P.'s on hair

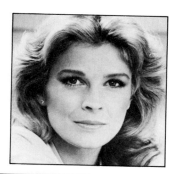

Candice Bergen:

Suga brings a new kind of order and artistry to hair—a certain Japanese sensibility and approach which extends naturally to all he does. He seems to know more than anyone about hair and what is appropriate for each person.

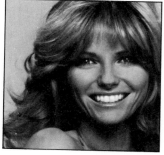

Cheryl Tiegs:

Getting the right haircut makes hair care easy and carefree. Frankly, the professional touch is essential. When I went to do the *Time* cover it was very important for me to think only of the shooting and not about hair. Thanks to Suga, it was possible to do just that.

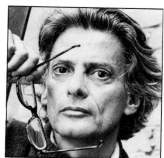

Richard Avedon:

Suga from the East is the fastest comb in the West.

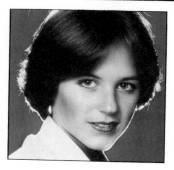

Dorothy Hamill:

Besides the fact that he is the sweetest, kindest, most adorable person I know, he must be doing something right. They call it the Dorothy Hamill haircut and lots of people are wearing it!

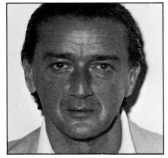

Victor Skrebneski:
Suga is an artist whose talent, skill and reputation enhance the fashion image of New York. It is always a pleasure to work with him.

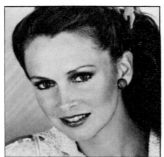

Karen Graham:
Suga helped me realize that hair shapes the face, accentuating the strong features and disguising the weak, making an ordinary girl into an eye catcher, or a good photograph into a smashing page stopper. Bottom line: Choose your hair stylist as though you were choosing a plastic surgeon. I did when I chose Suga.

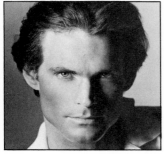

Joe MacDonald:
Suga's taught me when hair is properly cut you can just shake it into place. Since I've been to Suga I've thrown the blow-dryer away!

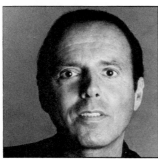

Francesco Scavullo:
I think the best look for hair is a fabulous cut. Hair should look great in bed, wet, in the wind, and at dinner. Suga understands these things.

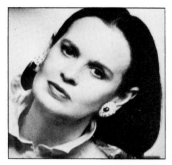

Gloria Vanderbilt:

As in fashion, I believe in a signature approach to hair. I've worn the same simple, straight styling for years and find no need to experiment with fads. This kind of look demands the best in regular haircuts, and Suga provides it.

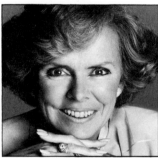

Eileen Ford:

Suga is a super hairstylist for superstars, models and society women—celebrities from all over the world would take the Concorde to New York rather than have anyone else cut their hair. There's nothing about hair he doesn't know and won't reveal to you in this book.

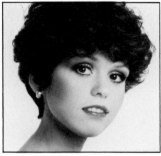

Marie Osmond:

Maintaining the look that suits you best is important, and finding a stylist who can help you obtain that look is just as important. I found mine in Suga.

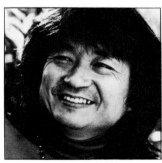

Seiji Ozawa:

My wife, Vera, introduced me to Mr. Suga a number of years ago in Tokyo. Although I am totally unconcerned about my appearance, Mr. Suga is nice enough to trim my messy mane whenever I'm in New York City, about twice a year, and Vera touches it up in between. The whole orchestra knows when we're in New York because I can see the back stands and look a lot neater!

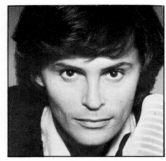

Way Bandy:
Suga is one of the greatest designers of hair style who have ever lived. To see him work with hair is to see a genius create.

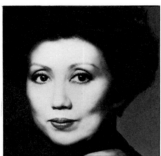

Hanae Mori:
The well-dressed woman realizes that hair is her most important accessory. I look personally and professionally to Suga for that enhancement.

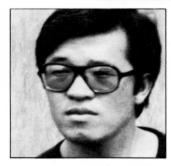

Hiro:
I've always felt Suga understands hair the way a great couturier understands fabric.

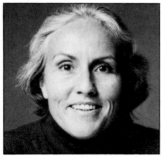

Polly Allen Mellen:
Knowing Suga has only been a plus in my working life at *Vogue.* To have him on a sitting has given me the freedom to do "my thing" because of my total confidence in him. He is a haircutter supreme. His understanding of a situation and care of a person's beauty is complete.

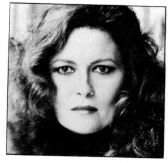

Faye Dunaway:

Suga to hair is like sushi to Japan, essential. He combines all the great skills of traditional maestros with a touch of simplicity, gentleness and a unique imagination that puts him in a class of his own.

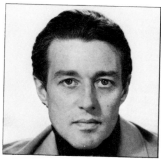

Halston:

Suga is one of the nicest and sweetest persons I know with a superb and unusual talent. He can do almost anything on every level as far as cutting and styling.

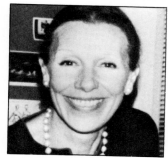

Françoise de la Renta:

Just a look at Suga gives you confidence and joy. He is probably the biggest expert on everything about hair: treatment, cut, or fantasy. I've known him for years, so I know what I am talking about.

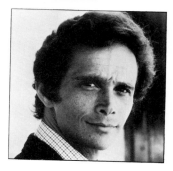

Joel Grey:

Suga has been cutting the "Grey" hair—my wife's, mine and our two children's—for a number of years. One never gets the feeling of a trendy style changing in anything he does; it has a sense of today, as well as a classic simplicity. One could say the same thing about Suga. He emanates a style that, like a pair of well-tailored gray flannel trousers, never dates and will always wear well.

Photo Credits

Candice Bergen: Vorkapich/"Cie"; Cheryl Tiegs: Hiro/*Time*; Dorothy Hamill: Bob Young/Ice Capades; Victor Skrebneski: Papadakis; Francesco Scavullo: Sean Byrnes; Gloria Vanderbilt: Duane Michaels; Eileen Ford: Scavullo; Seiji Ozawa: Uli Markle; Way Bandy: Al Levine; Hanae Mori: Hiro; Polly Allen Mellen: Jeff Niki; Faye Dunaway: Terry O'Neill

Index